WATCH YO

A Quality of

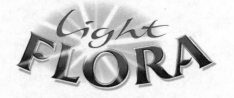

WATCH YOUR WEIGHT

A Quality of Life Approach

DR GILLIAN MOORE-GROARKE

&

TERESA NERNEY

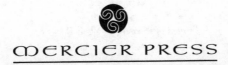

MERCIER PRESS

MERCIER PRESS
Douglas Village, Cork
www.mercierpress.ie

Trade enquiries to COLUMBA MERCIER DISTRIBUTION,
55a Spruce Avenue, Stillorgan Industrial Park, Blackrock, Dublin

© Dr Gillian Moore-Groarke & Teresa Nerney

ISBN: 1 85635 433 4

10 9 8 7 6 5 4 3 2 1

DEDICATED TO JAYNE

Printed in Ireland by Colour Books Ltd

Contents

Acknowledgements   7
Preface by Dr Aileen McGloin   9
   Consultant Nutritionist to Flora Light
Foreword by Rita Fagan   11
   Managing Director Weight Watchers Ireland
Authors' Note   13

Step 1

1 Getting to Know Yourself   18
2 Finding the Evidence   23

Step 2

3 Seeing Things as They Are   30
4 Believing You Can Do It   36

Step 3

5 Conquering Your Fears   44
6 Riding Life's Roller Coaster   52

Step 4

7 Getting to Where You Want to Be   60
8 Daring to Imagine   67

Step 5

9   Finding Out if You are Really Hungry   76

Step 6

10 Sharing Your Dream   88
11 Reclaiming Your Rights   98

Step 7

12 Creating a New Life   104
13 Staying Slim for Life   115

Appendix: Useful Names and Addresses   122
Progress Chart   124
Recommended Reading   127

Acknowledgements

To all who helped in various ways with this book, we would like to say 'thank you', particularly Colette O'Brien of *Flora Light*, Gina Jones of Wilson Hartnell Public Relations, Rita Fagan and Carmel Smith of *Weight Watchers Ireland*, and Mary Feehan and John Spillane of Mercier Press.

A personal word of thanks from Gillian:
To my husband James, and wonderful daughter Jayne, my parents Anne and John for their love, support and encouragement along the path of life. A special word of thanks to my colleagues and secretary Deirdre Cashman for her ongoing dedication and support.

A personal word of thanks from Teresa:
To my parents John Joe and Agnes and my family for all their support over the years, and to the following people who were a great help to me: Mary Finn, Eilish Talbot and Chris O'Gara. Finally, special thanks to my husband, Séamus, who was with me, as always, every step of the way.

Preface by Flora Light

The key to healthy, sustained weight loss is having a healthy positive attitude along with balanced, healthy living.

The fact is that fad diets don't work. They may give you a quick-fix weight loss but you're not going to be able to stick to them forever, so as soon as you return to your old habits, the weight will just pile back on.

Nutritionists have always advocated that a few simple lifestyle changes can lead to long-term results, maintaining a healthy weight, helping to keep your heart healthy and making you look and feel great! That means enjoying a little of what you fancy in moderation rather than depriving yourself of those foods you enjoy. That way you'll keep your motivation high *and* deliver long-term results.

Losing weight needn't be an uphill struggle – if you set yourself smaller, more manageable goals then long term weight loss can be well within your reach – remember, you *can* do it!

Don't forget to allow yourself the occasional reward – when you need a treat, don't run to the fridge – give yourself a new CD, a trip to the movies, or maybe a new pair of earrings instead. By rewarding yourself every time you reach a milestone in your weight loss programme, you're reinforcing your success, adding to your own sense of achievement and boosting your self-confidence.

This book can help you on the road to successful weight loss and *Flora Light* is delighted to be a part of that journey. Healthy weight loss is easier than you think. With a few small lifestyle changes and a bit of good fun exercise thrown in, you'll be astonished at the results – and they'll last a lifetime!

Best of luck!

Dr Aileen McGloin
Consultant Nutritionist to Flora Light

Foreword

Over the last twenty-five years working with *Weight Watchers*, I have witnessed thousands of members come through our doors, some who successfully managed to lose weight and some who unfortunately did not.

It has always been a source of fascination to me, why some people achieve their weight loss goal so easily, making a dramatic lifestyle change in the process, while for others it is a continuous struggle.

The difference, of course, lies in the attitudes and belief-system that people bring with them into our meeting rooms. The simple key to successful weight loss is to eat less and exercise more, yet if it really is this straightforward then why are there so many people out there who just cannot seem to achieve a healthy weight?

The answer is that weight is not just a physical issue, we are emotional beings and it is within this realm the solution to a weight problem is to be found. By simply acknowledging that being overweight is more tied up with how we think and feel than what we eat, we have already made a huge stride towards conquering the problem. It is for this reason that for those who are ready to honestly review and re-evaluate their thought process before tackling a weight issue, success is almost guaranteed.

This book, by addressing these emotional and psychological issues, targets the very roots of obesity, an approach that offers a unique insight.

Both authors are eminently placed to guide the reader through his or her weight loss journey. Dr Gillian, through her work has made incredible strides in helping people to achieve and maintain a healthy weight and as a consultant to *Weight Watchers*, has also proved an invaluable source of information into human behaviour. Teresa Nerney has always written with great empathy and sensitivity about those with a weight problem and has a great understanding of all the issues dealt with in this book; she has first hand knowledge and understanding of the practical challenges that people encounter on a day-to-day basis.

It is, therefore, without hesitation that I recommend this book to those who are on a journey of self-discovery.

RITA FAGAN
Managing Director
Weight Watchers Ireland

Authors' Note

It's easy to put on weight, to settle for the next dress size up, the extra notch in the belt. But why settle for a less healthy life? Many of us do so, however, because we think we are unable to lose weight. At one stage or another we have given up and told ourselves something like the following:

There's no point in dieting – my Monday morning plans always fizzle out. I'm just no good at it!

Someday, I will eat healthily, but not today because I'm too busy, I'm too tired, I'm not in a good mood ...

I don't see the benefit of going to all that trouble to lose weight when I know I will pile it all back on again. I might as well enjoy my food, despite the consequences.

Other people are able to lose weight but not me. They have more will-power than me because they're not as busy as me, they're more confident than me, they don't have as much weight to lose as me ...

This book helps you understand that losing weight is possible, that *you can do it*! We help you understand why, in the past, your attempts at weight loss have failed and we give you the tools to succeed this time round. Losing weight is a challenge and we will not tell you otherwise, but it really is worth the effort, as every successful slimmer knows.

For the past 14 years, Dr Gillian Moore-Groarke has shared first-hand the joys and disappointments of people in their attempts to lose weight and keep it off. Teresa Nerney, in documenting the triumphs of members of *Weight Watchers Ireland*, has interviewed countless men and women about their weight loss experiences.

Those who succeed describe the experience as extremely pleasurable, rewarding, exciting and fulfilling. They talk about themselves in terms of 'a new person' and develop a positive outlook on life. They look forward to healthy eating plans and regular exercise routines. They learn to take better care of themselves, improve their self-esteem, address their everyday needs and, very importantly, start to relax. They say they never realised how much their weight was holding them back.

On the other hand, those who don't succeed, experience conflict, disappointment and frustration as they struggle with yo-yo dieting, starvation, detox plans, and the many other fad diets and gimmicks on the market nowadays.

Losing weight for life is about making permanent lifestyle changes and to do this we need, first of all, to become aware of what we are telling ourselves. We need to confront that nagging negative voice in our heads that tells us we're no good at dieting, that it may work for other people but not for us, that we are not strong enough to stick to our healthy living plan and so on.

That is why this book starts with *you*. The bottom line is that you need to make the correct choices, so we promote a pro-active involvement by you. In completing the exercises in each chapter, you become aware of the innermost thoughts, feelings and beliefs that are keeping you in the weight trap. Therefore, you play an active part in your own recovery.

HOW TO USE THIS BOOK

This book contains a 7-step plan, which gives you the tools to prepare mentally and emotionally to lose weight and improve the quality of your life. We recommend that you use this plan in conjunction with a healthy weight loss and exercise programme.

• It is best to work through the book, beginning at Step 1 and concluding at Step 7. Don't expect to read it at thriller speed, don't be tempted to dip into it or, dare we say, read from the back! Complete all the exercises at your own pace, there's no benefit in rushing through chapters, skipping over exercises or taking on our suggestions all at once. Take each step one at a time and set yourself one goal at a time. If you try to do too much too quickly, you will achieve less.

- In each chapter, you will find exercises to complete and sometimes there will be homework to do. This allows *you* to play a very real part in your own weight loss – *you are always in the driving seat*. You will need to buy yourself a diary or notebook in which to chart your progress; this can double-up as a reference for your own personal notes.

- At the end of each step, we provide *tools for action*, a brief reminder of what you need to do before you progress to the next step.

- In the appendix (pp. 125–126), there is a *progress chart* where you can map your weight loss as you move through the book, as well as a list of useful names and addresses should you require further assistance.

This book is your practical resource as you prepare for a healthier life, as well as your reference as you journey towards weight loss with the support of a healthy eating and exercise programme. Within these pages you will learn that, just like every other successful slimmer, *you can lose weight*, keep it off and enrich the quality of your life.

A good philosophy to bear in mind is that we are born crying, we live complaining and if we are not careful, we will die disappointed, having never conquered the dreaded weight trap. What a waste that would be, so let *now* be your time for action!

I tried to lose weight several times but it never seemed to work. If I did manage to lose weight, I would just put it all back again. I reckon I'm just no good at dieting.

STEP 1

UNDERSTAND WHY YOU ARE NOT A HEALTHY WEIGHT NOW

1

Getting to Know Yourself

The focus of this book is not food, but how you can prepare mentally and emotionally to successfully lose weight and keep it off. If you are ready to lose weight in your head, then you will be able to do it with the help of a healthy weight loss programme combined with regular gentle exercise. *We slim from the inside out.*

Firstly, we recommend that you consult your general practitioner for a thorough medical examination before you embark on a weight loss and exercise programme. Your doctor will know your medical history and will advise accordingly. S/he will weigh you and suggest a healthy target weight using the Body Mass Index (BMI) method, internationally recognised as the most accurate way to calculate healthy weights for individuals. (The BMI chart on page 19 gives you an indication of what is a healthy weight for you.)

For some, the journey may warrant additional professional help, for example there may be issues in your childhood that have contributed to your unhealthy relationship with food and in this case, it may be helpful to attend a qualified psychologist or counsellor. In the appendix, you will find a list of organisations that will help you follow a sensible eating and exercise programme as well as a list of organisations that will give you guidance if you need to consult a qualified psychologist or counsellor.

Body Mass Index Chart – Healthy Weight Range
Body Mass Index is the ratio of weight to height squared (your weight in kilogrammes divided by the square of your height in metres). The four BMI classifications – normal, healthy weight (BMI 20 – 24.9); over-

$$BMI = \frac{weight\ [kg]}{height^2\ [m^2]}$$

weight (BMI 25 – 29.9); obese (BMI 30 – 39.9), and very obese (40 and over). The following chart indicates what is a normal, healthy weight based on height.

As stated previously, we recommend that you consult your general practitioner before setting your target weight and embarking on a weight loss plan. For example, your doctor may advise that first of all, you aim to lose 10% of your body weight – whether this reduction brings you within the healthy BMI range or not, it will most definitely result in noticeable health benefits.

The following abbreviations apply: ft = foot, ins = inches, m = metres, st = stone, lbs = pounds, kgs = kilograms

HEIGHT	BMI 20 – 24.9
	(Normal, healthy weight for men and women)
4 ft 10 ins	**6 st 12 lbs – 8 st 8 lbs**
1.47 m	43.2 kgs – 54.0 kgs
4 ft 11 ins	**7 st 1 lb – 8 st 12 lbs**
1.50 m	45.0 kgs – 56.2 kgs
5 ft 0 ins	**7 st 4 lbs – 9 st 2 lbs**
1.52 m	46.2 kgs – 57.8 kgs
5 ft 1 ins	**7 st 8 lbs – 9 st 6 lbs**
1.55 m	48.0 kgs – 60.0 kgs
5 ft 2 ins	**7 st 11 lbs – 9 st 11 lbs**
1.57 m	49.4 kgs – 61.6 kgs
5 ft 3 ins	**8 st 1 lb – 10 st 1 lb**
1.60 m	51.2 kgs – 64.0 kgs
5 ft 4 ins	**8 st 5 lbs – 10 st 6 lbs**
1.63 m	53.2 kgs – 66.4 kgs
5 ft 5 ins	**8 st 8 lbs – 10 st 10 lbs**
1.65 m	54.4 kgs – 68.0 kgs
5 ft 6 ins	**8 st 12 lbs – 11 st 1 lb**
1.68 m	56.4 kgs – 70.6 kgs
5 ft 7 ins	**9 st 2 lbs – 11 st 6 lbs**
1.70 m	57.8 kgs – 72.2 kgs
5 ft 8 ins	**9 st 6 lbs – 11 st 10 lbs**
1.73 m	59.8 kgs – 74.8 kgs

5 ft 9 ins	**9 st 9 lbs – 12 st 1 lb**
1.75 m	61.2 kgs – 76.6 kgs
5 ft 10 ins	**9 st 13 lbs – 12 st 6 lbs**
1.78 m	63.4 kgs – 79.2 kgs
5 ft 11 ins	**10 st 3 lbs – 12 st 11 lbs**
1.80 m	64.8 kgs – 81.0 kgs
6 ft	**10 st 7 lbs – 13 st 2 lbs**
1.83 m	67.0 kgs – 83.8 kgs
6 ft 1 in	**10 st 12 lbs – 13 st 7 lbs**
1.85 m	68.4 kgs – 85.6 kgs
6 ft 2 ins	**11 st 2 lbs – 13 st 13 lbs**
1.88 m	70.6 kgs – 88.4 kgs

The BMI table is used courtesy of Weight Watchers

Progress chart

After you have committed to following a healthy eating and exercise programme with proper dietary education and advice, turn to page 126 and use the progress chart to map your weight loss as you move through this book.

Making your escape from the weight trap

Have you ever wondered why you struggle with your weight? Why every time you plan to go on a diet, you end up eating twice the amount you normally eat? Why every time you do manage to lose a few pounds, you give up and put them all back on again? By now you may be living with your extra weight even though you know it is putting a strain on your physical and psychological health. What a pity, because this means you are not enjoying life as much as you could be.

First of all, remember that nobody sets out to be overweight, so stop blaming yourself! For many people, the pounds just creep up on them. One day they were slim and active, then maybe they bought their first car and put on a few pounds which they never bothered to lose. Another lifestyle change occurred, maybe they moved job and were under a lot of pressure and, before they knew it, the pounds had turned into stones.

Now they're overweight and feeling bad about themselves. They become stressed and fed up, internalising negative thoughts and feelings, and the end result can be depression. This, in turn, leads to further patterns of overeating and then the continuous cycle of overeating. When we add factors that contribute to weight increase, and our personality types, combined with perhaps a family history of depression, or depression as a reaction to stress/anxiety or trauma, we become even more enmeshed in the weight trap.

Diagrammatically it looks something like this:

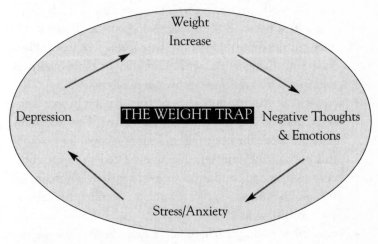

The weight trap is a vicious cycle in which weight increase leads to negative thoughts and emotions, which causes stress/anxiety, and, if this stress/anxiety is not addressed, a further reactive depression results. This, in turn, increases weight even more and the whole cycle begins all over again.

Now is the time to make your escape from the weight trap and take care of *you*. In the next chapter, we help you identify the false beliefs that are, ultimately, holding you back from achieving your weight loss dreams.

Homework: create your own image file

- Dust down your photograph albums and ask somebody close to help you pick out photographs of yourself at different ages, from baby to present day. Don't just pick out the ones you like, pick out the ones you don't like as well. You must confront the ones you are unhappy with too, for instance when you became overweight, you may have tried to hide at the back of groups to disguise your weight, so pick out these photos as well.

- Think about each of the photographs you have chosen and how you felt at that stage in your life. If as a teenager, you looked slim and healthy, ask yourself what was going on in your life at that time. Try to remember how you felt about yourself. What were the thoughts in your head? What has changed since then? How have your feelings changed? How have your thoughts changed? Think about these questions and write down the answers in your notebook.

- Now pick out your favourite photograph and put it in your notebook. Why do you like this one in particular? What does it represent? Write the key words in your notebook, for example this photo could represent happiness, freedom, confidence, optimism, and so on. Each time you open your notebook, let this photo remind you of what you are working towards on your path to weight loss.

- Some people find it helpful to take a new photo of themselves so that they can face up to how they look now and how much they want to change their image. When they have reached their goal weight, the contrast between the before and after picture helps them keep in mind how much they have achieved.

- If you have no photos of yourself, then cut out a picture of somebody you admire and use that instead. *A word of caution here:* choose somebody who carries a normal healthy weight, rather than somebody who is significantly underweight. Your aim is to achieve a healthy weight loss, not an unhealthy one.

2

Finding the Evidence

It is a fact of physics that any ingested calories not used are stored. In other words, if we eat more food than our bodies use in energy, we put on weight. Maintaining a healthy weight means eating the right amount of food to supply our energy needs. Sounds so simple doesn't it?

However, we are complex human beings with fundamental beliefs about ourselves, which influence how we think, feel and behave. Some of us, as we move through life, start to believe a lot of negative things and each time our performance falls short of perfect these beliefs are further reinforced. Indeed, we could be carrying around a whole portfolio of negativity without any evidence to back it up! Most of the time, we are not aware that this is happening until we become unhappy with a particular issue such as our weight.

In the case of our weight, our belief system is portrayed in the way we treat our bodies. If we have a poor belief system, then we enter a traumatic battleground of never feeling worthy enough to tackle the weight trap. Each new quick-fix trick at losing weight inspires less confidence in ourselves in the long run, and we file more evidence in our portfolio to support the negative belief. To lose weight successfully, we need to learn to believe:

I am a worthwhile person.

If you believe you are a worthwhile person, you believe you deserve to be healthy and make the most of your life. You believe you can achieve weight loss, and with this belief, *you will*. When you lapse along the way, as everybody does, you will not give yourself a hard time for failing, but your inner belief in your own worth will help you pick up the pieces and start again.

So, if you do not believe at this present moment that you are a worthwhile person, how do you start believing it? First of all, you need to prove that your negative thoughts are not based on truth. In changing our thoughts, we change how we feel and behave.

All our emotions – fear, anger, sadness, anxiety, jealousy, depression – are a physical response to our thoughts. When it comes to weight loss, anger and fear are our strongest emotions – anger, if we turn it in on ourselves, leads to destructive behaviour; fear holds us back from our goals. Like every other emotion, you can transform these emotions by choosing to let your thought processes work with you as opposed to against you:

Thoughts

Feelings

Behaviour

Changing how we think is, therefore, the key to changing how we feel and behave.

☺ *Happy Face = Positive Inner Voice*

☹ *Sad Face = Negative Inner Voice*

We all use inner speech but negative self-talk can be replaced to reinforce positive behaviour patterns.

Confronting our negative thoughts is not something we normally do, so you may find it difficult at first to assess how your

NAME YOUR NEGATIVE VOICE

Get in control of your thoughts by giving the negative inner voice a name. This way, every time you hear it, you will instantly recognise and confront it. The name we have chosen is Dot the Distorter because this voice literally distorts the way we think – when the least little thing goes wrong, it makes us think everything is pear-shaped. If you wish to use another name, feel free to do so, as long as the name you choose helps you become aware of the negative things you are telling yourself.

- *Every time Dot the Distorter tells you that you can't lose weight, tell it you can.*
- *Every time Dot the Distorter tells you there's no point in dieting, tell it there is.*
- *Every time Dot the Distorter tells you that you are a failure, tell it that's not true and recall all you have achieved in life.*

In your notebook, list your positive and negative thoughts every day and at the end of each week, add up the number of positive and negative thoughts. Aim to reduce the number of negative thoughts the following week. It will be interesting to see how your new way of thinking will help you in the long run. By asking yourself, how can I replace each negative thought with a positive thought you are further working on the Getting to Know You process.

thoughts are affecting your feelings and behaviour. Here are some Dos and Don'ts when trying to change your thinking process:

- Do be patient with yourself. Don't expect to be able to think and feel positively instantly. Remember, you probably have been thinking and feeling negatively for quite some time.
- If your negative thoughts and feelings continue to recur, don't be discouraged. Just keep looking for the evidence to prove them wrong.
- Don't believe your negative voice when it calls you a failure

just because your healthy eating plan falls short of perfect. This type of all-or-nothing thinking will make you feel even worse.

- When recording your negative thoughts and feelings, do bear in mind that raising your awareness of them is a very positive step, so don't be critical of yourself.

Homework: challenge Dot the Distorter
Record your thoughts and feelings so that you become aware of how crippling negative thinking can be when trying to achieve a weight loss goal. We provide you with two examples of how to challenge Dot the Distorter, and using this question and answer formula, you can do the same whenever you encounter a situation where your thinking is causing you to feel bad.

You will discover that when you replace a negative thought with a positive one, you will feel a lot better. By continually challenging your negative thought processes, you are chipping away at your false inner beliefs, such as I am an unworthy person, I don't deserve to lose weight, and so on. Eventually, as you start to think more positively and feel better about yourself (and this will only happen gradually), the positive beliefs will outweigh the negative.

Example No. 1

What is Dot the Distorter telling me?
I might as well give up dieting.

How does this make me feel?
Angry and guilty.

Is what Dot the Distorter says based on truth?
Well, I did lapse from my healthy eating programme this morning.

What is Dot the Distorter not telling me?
I have been doing really well. I have been eating healthily for over a week now.

What will I tell Dot the Distorter now?
One lapse is no problem – I'm only human after all. I can start again now.

How does this make me feel now?
More confident that I can start again.

Example No. 2

What is Dot the Distorter telling me?
I have a lot of work to do and I don't think I can cope with dieting.

How does this make me feel?
Anxious and tired.

Is what Dot the Distorter says based on truth?
Last time I was stressed at work, I did overeat and gave up my diet.

What is Dot the Distorter not telling me?
I've had other stresses since I started eating healthily and I stuck to my diet.

What will I tell Dot the Distorter now?
I can do other things to help me cope with my workload – go for a massage, go for a walk.

How does this make me feel now?
More in control of my weight loss plan.

Now fill in your own answers:

What is Dot the Distorter telling me?

_____

How does this make me feel?

_____

Is what Dot the Distorter says based on truth?

_____

What is Dot the Distorter not telling me?

_____

What will I tell Dot the Distorter now?

_____

How does this make me feel now?

_____

☞ *Tools for action*

You have come to the end of Step 1 on your journey to permanent weight loss, where we have given you the tools to *understand why you are not a healthy weight now.*

Here is a reminder of what you need to do before you progress to Step 2.

• Seek the advice of your doctor before you embark on a weight loss and exercise programme. H/she will advise about how much weight you need to lose to stay healthy.

• Follow a sensible programme that educates you about eating and exercising for your health. Record your weight loss by using the progress chart as you move through the book.

• Become aware of how much your negative thinking is keeping you stuck in the weight trap.

• Change what you believe about yourself by challenging your negative thinking.

I knew I was putting on more weight all the time, so I started buying baggy tops and trousers with elastic waist bands, and I tried to pretend to myself that I still looked slim.

STEP 2

FACE UP TO THE FACT THAT YOU NEED TO LOSE WEIGHT

3

Seeing Things as They Are

The choice to lose weight is yours and yours alone. Your doctor may advise you, family and friends may encourage you, but at the end of the day nobody can force you to lose weight and no weight loss programme will work if *you* do not really want to lose weight.

Seeing things as they are means taking responsibility for being overweight, and the more responsibility you take for your own body, the greater strength of mind you will have to work towards changing it. Granted, your circumstances may have contributed to your weight problem, but there's no point in blaming others or playing the role of victim. Nothing will change unless you make it change.

To help you make the choice to lose weight for life, the following is a contract we suggest you make with yourself:

I AGREE THAT:

I am responsible for what I eat.
The choice to eat healthily is mine.
Nobody is forcing me to overeat.
My body reflects how I approach food.
I can choose to change how I look and to take better care of myself.

Signed _____ *Dated* _____

As you progress though this book and follow the exercises we recommend, you will begin to know yourself better and understand how you can play a proactive role in your own weight loss.

It's a good idea, therefore, to review your contract after each step of this book.

Putting your health in focus
When we use food responsibly, eating can be one of life's most enjoyable experiences. Just think, isn't there something wonderful about sharing an intimate meal with friends? However, if we overeat to the detriment of our health, our eating habits become problematic. This is evident from global overweight and obesity levels.

While it's easy enough to hide excess weight under baggy tops and stretchy trousers, it's much more difficult to ignore the alarm bells that tell you your health is at risk. When out of breath at the top of stairs just because of the excess weight you're carrying, or unable to keep up with the children because your weight is slowing you down, it's time to face up to the fact that *you need to start losing weight before you start suffering serious ill health!*

Here are some of the physical health problems linked to overweight and obesity:

- Arthritis – particularly hips and knees
- Cirrhosis of the liver
- Constipation and bowel disorder
- Dental decay
- Diabetes and its complications
- Fatigue
- Gallstone problems
- Heart disease
- High blood cholesterol
- Hypertension (high blood pressure) – increases risk of coronary heart disease and stroke
- Impotence/ Infertility
- Kidney stones
- Rheumatism

- Poor lung function – shortness of breath
- Varicose Veins

You now need to consider – are you prepared to suffer serious ill health because of your weight?

Recognising how different life could be
The weighing scales indicate you're overweight but you still have difficulty facing up to the fact that you need to shed those pounds. How about getting somebody to take a photo of you? When you see this photograph, become aware of how you react. What do you see? What are you avoiding seeing?

Take this exercise a step further by standing in front of full-length mirror the next time you step out of the shower. Look at yourself. Do you like what you see? This may be difficult but ask yourself, how long have you been in denial that you need to lose weight?

Whether you like what you see or not, please don't criticise yourself. You are a human being whose body deserves to be treated with respect. Do not loathe the way you look but love and respect your body and acknowledge that no matter what size you are, your body has still served you well. It has afforded you the opportunity to work, perhaps have children, to give and receive love, and more.

Out of *love for yourself*, decide now to choose to take care of your body, to lose weight so that you feel better physically. This way you are ensuring that your body will continue to serve you well.

Lucy's Story

Lucy is a 35-year-old mother of two and 3 stone overweight. She says that her weight is affecting her health, relationships and happiness. Like Lucy, you may find that the extra pounds you are carrying are having a negative impact on many areas of your life.

'I had my second child, Frank, two years ago and am still carrying the weight I gained during pregnancy, plus more. I just never managed to lose any of it. For the first few months after he was born, I felt really tired and stressed. My sleeping pattern was all over the place and I just ended up eating lots of chocolate and sugary food just to keep myself perked up. But I never really gained more energy in the long-term. I still feel tired most of the time. It's an effort to push the buggy when I'm shopping. The doctor told me I needed to do something about my weight before it became more of a problem for me.

'I have a great husband and two beautiful children, but sometimes I feel if I had more energy, I would be able to do more things with them. I rarely play with my eldest son, James, because I'm not able to keep up with him. I just end up being out of breath and feeling really uncomfortable even when we're only kicking a ball around the garden.

'People look at me and think I am so lucky to have a great family, a beautiful house and a job I love, but sometimes I feel so unhappy inside. I really dislike the way I look since I put on weight and I hate the fact that I don't seem able to do something about it. I hate going shopping for clothes now and when I do go out at night, I feel inadequate beside other people. I feel I don't look good and I don't really enjoy myself.'

In your notebook, write about yourself at this present moment. Ask yourself, in what way does your extra weight affect your everyday life, your relationships and your health. Afterwards, take some time out to think about how much your life would change if you lost weight. Write down at least one change. For example, it might be that you would no longer have problems when shopping for trendy, figure-hugging clothes. Keep this in mind every time you feel like giving up.

Learning to love you and your food
You probably have heard the following statement (or maybe said it yourself): 'I love food too much to give it up'. Many people who struggle with their weight imagine that eating healthily means denying themselves the pleasure of food. However, when following a balanced diet, you do not give food up or stop enjoying it, in fact, you savour food even more and, as your taste buds change, discover all kinds of new food experiences.

Get in tune with your relationship with food by answering 'Yes' or 'No' to the following questions:

1 Do you like to pick at food rather than allow yourself to become really hungry?
2 Would you rather eat bread and jam (or some other snack) instantly, rather than wait half an hour for a proper meal?
3 Do you sometimes have your mouth so full it is difficult to chew?
4 Do you prefer to eat alone because you don't want other people knowing how much you eat?
5 Do you eat left-overs even though you are not hungry?
6 Have you ever had more than three different clothes sizes at any one time (apart from pregnancy)?
7 When you are supermarket shopping, do you always have to buy something 'nice' to eat for now or when you get home?
8 Would you find it harder to give up chocolate than a close friend?

If you answer 'Yes' to five or more of these questions, you need to consider changing your eating habits and moving towards a healthier lifestyle.

Homework: Nutrition counselling questionnaire

In changing your eating habits, it is important to let go of your old relationship with food. By answering this Nutrition Counselling Questionnaire, you will become aware of the eating patterns you have developed over the years and identify the areas where greater control is needed:

1 What foods did you eat growing up?
    (a) Which foods did you like?
    (b) Which foods did you dislike?

2 Which of those foods do you still eat?
    (a) Something you hated that you eat now?
    (b) Something you like you don't eat now?

3 Which foods were special treats?
    (a) What activities and people were involved?
    (b) How do you feel about those foods then and now?

4 How else has your diet changed?
    (a) What is your diet like now?

5 What would you like to change about your diet?

4

Believing You Can Do It

'You are what you believe you are and you can become what you believe you can become' – these were the words of one of Dr Moore-Groarke's patients, and how right she was. When you believe that you can lose weight ...

√ You take positive action to control your eating habits.
√ You explore all the options available and make informed choices.
√ You learn to love yourself even when you don't get everything right.
√ You persist until your weight loss programme becomes part of your new lifestyle.
√ You set your spirit free from the fear and despair in which the weight trap ensnares you.

Along the way, there will be several temptations. We call these the doors that you choose not to open. Later, we will help you identify these temptations by helping you understand what triggers you to overeat. Meantime, take the following into consideration:

• What will self-belief do for you as far as your eating habits are concerned?
• How will believing in yourself make you feel?
• What things will it allow you to do with your life?
• What are its long-term benefits?
• How will your new body change you?
• How will it make you feel?

• What more will it enable you to do and feel?

Here is a list of self-limiting, negative beliefs that keep us stuck in the weight trap. Do any of them sound familiar to you?

    ✗ I am no good. Others are better.
    ✗ I am not worth loving.
    ✗ I hate myself.
    ✗ I don't deserve success.
    ✗ My life is such a struggle every day.
    ✗ My life has had so many disappointments.

Now try to take control of these statements by changing each one to a positive one.

√ I am creative in all that I do.
√ I feel loved by my friends and family.
√ I can learn to love myself.
√ I deserve success when I make an effort in my life.
√ Life today was good for me.
√ I did not feel disappointed with my achievements today.

Your next exercise is to list all the excuses you have ever made in the past for avoiding weight loss. Spend some time writing them down and again replace all these excuses with positive, self-controlling statements that guide you towards the process of change.

Weeding out the enemy
Remember Dot the Distorter who tells us 'we can't' and 'we won't' be able to achieve our goals. Control this enemy within and keep reinforcing yourself with positive affirmations.

    Here are some examples of affirmations that will help:

I love and respect my body
I love my life and a good quality of life
I balance my positive and negative sides
I am at peace with myself
I accept my individuality
I am a worthwhile person and people love me

Homework: Create your own personality file
In Chapter 2, we showed you how negative thinking causes us to feel and behave negatively. Here we ask you to create your own personality profile by listing the positive and negative aspects of your personality. We provide you with an example of personality traits to help you understand how they can influence weight loss. Once again, by changing the way we think we can also work on swapping our negative personality traits for positive ones.

DOs and DON'TS for personality profile
- None of us have perfect personalities, so be as honest as possible and don't avoid listing some negative traits.
- Don't criticise yourself when listing your negative personality traits. This is an exercise in self-awareness, not in self-criticism. By becoming aware of the traits that are interfering with your weight loss plan, you are making a very important step in the process of self-change.
- Do seek help and advice from people who love you. They will help you take a long, hard look at yourself without passing judgement.
- Once you have completed this part of the exercise, do try to apply each positive and negative trait to your weight loss plan. Draw on the personality traits which will help you with weight loss and become aware of those which won't. Awareness will eventually help you control and change these traits.

POSITIVE TRAITS	NEGATIVE TRAITS
Patient – you accept slow and regular weight loss.	*Envious – you can't enjoy other people's successes because you measure your success against theirs. Tell yourself that your success is as individual as you are.*
Flexible – you are willing to change your habits so that you will lose weight.	*Angry – you feel angry with yourself and the world that you are overweight. Challenge your negative thoughts so that you do not become bitter and self-absorbed.*
Helpful – you are not afraid to ask for help to reach your goal.	*Moody – you have good and bad moods and when they're bad, you overeat and lapse from your healthy eating plan. Change your moods by changing the way you think and, therefore, react.*
Confident – you believe in yourself and know that you can succeed at losing weight.	*Perfectionist – you want your weight loss to be perfect. Therefore, you either never try to lose weight in case your performance falls short of perfect, or you give up after the first attempt. Accept that nobody is perfect, not even you, otherwise you will never be happy with yourself.*
Modest – you are happy with yourself, warts and all. Therefore, you are gentle with yourself and others.	*Sponge-like – you are very influenced by what other people think and say, and your actions are swayed accordingly. A simple comment such as, 'You don't need to lose weight, you are fine'*

the way you are', is enough to make you not lose weight. Learn to think for yourself or you will always be trying to please other people, solve their problems and end up neglecting yourself.

Realistic – you know that you are not perfect so you pace yourself on your weight loss journey and strive for attainable goals.

Fearful – you are afraid to change because you are used to things the way they are. You might be stuck in a rut but you feel a certain comfort there. Changing means taking risks and you are afraid of what might happen. Understand that your fears will hold you back forever from your weight loss dreams unless you challenge them.

My personality profile

POSITIVE TRAITS	NEGATIVE TRAITS

☞ *Tools for action*

You have come to end of Step 2 on your journey to weight loss where you are learning to *face up to the fact that you need to lose weight*.

The following is a reminder of your *tools for action* before you progress to the next step.

√ Take responsibility for the fact you are overweight. Your life-style will not change unless you choose to change.

√ Answer this question honestly: Are you prepared to suffer serious ill health because of your weight?

√ Recognise that your life would be better if you were a healthy weight. Love your body, and out of love decide to take care of it.

√ Identify your eating habits and become aware of the areas where greater control is needed.

√ Believe you can lose weight and you will.

√ Work on swapping your negative personality traits for positive ones by learning to think positively.

I used to sit in the corner of the pub when we went out, and I never would get up for a dance. I just thought people would look at me and think, isn't she fat?

STEP 3

TAKE THE GAMBLE THAT YOU WILL SUCCEED

5

Conquering Your Fears

It's easy to opt out when overweight. Opt out of doing things, going places, meeting people. This way you imagine you are protecting yourself from all kinds of painful feelings – feeling inferior when you meet someone slim and confident, feeling embarrassed when you have to stand up in front of colleagues, or feeling self-conscious when you wear a new outfit.

Take a moment to consider these questions:

- Are you confident in social situations?
- Do you make friends easily?
- Do you have negative beliefs about yourself which prevent you from doing the things you want to do, letting your true self shine?

Say you go to a friend's wedding. You think everyone else looks better than you do and because of this negative thought you feel inadequate. You find it difficult to talk to people because you are comparing yourself to how they look. You don't enjoy the meal because you don't want people to think you overeat. When the music starts, you sit in the corner rather than get up on the dance floor because you think you look fat. In the end, you leave the wedding early and go home feeling down.

The natural reaction when we experience pain in a particular situation is to avoid ever getting into that situation again. If we had a difficult experience in the past when socialising, chances are we would be tempted to avoid socialising again because we anticipate a repeat of the experience. We persuade ourselves that we feel comfortable hanging around the house, renting a video and getting a pizza delivery.

Meanwhile, life goes on but we are at a standstill, living in the shadows, outsiders looking at life as if we are at the movies. We see other people going about, doing things, getting places and we are immobilised by feelings of powerlessness. We wonder how they do it with such apparent ease and why we can't. We fool ourselves into thinking we are shielding ourselves from pain by avoiding painful situations; the truth is that our inaction is causing even more pain. Our comfort zone turns out to be extremely uncomfortable!

> 'I was embarrassed about my weight, I hated going out,' Samantha recalled. 'When my husband wanted me to go out and meet his colleagues from work, I would make excuses. I'd say something like, 'I feel tired, I'm going to skip the meal tonight. You don't mind, do you?' Or I'd pretend to be really helpful and offer to look after the kids and tell him to go out and enjoy himself. I didn't really want to go out. I was just trying to fool him and myself. When I really had to go to something, like a family celebration, I would spend days deciding what to wear. In the end, I'd have worked myself into a complete state about the outfit, constantly seeking reassurance that I looked okay, but still having a sinking feeling every time I looked in the mirror.'

Samantha went on to lose five stone and, needless to say, today she has a completely different outlook on life. 'Now I'm the one who wants to go out all the time because I just feel so much better about myself!'

If you think your life would be a lot better if you were a healthy weight, what's stopping you from achieving weight loss? Why are you putting weight loss on the long finger? Could it be your fear of failure?

Replacing 'what if' with 'so what'

> 'Courage is resistance to fear, mastery of fear – not absence
> of fear' – Mark Twain.

We all have fears that we are aware of and many more subtle every-day fears we don't even notice. If you ask a person who appears confident how they manage not to be afraid, you will discover that they have fears too. The difference is that they choose not to let these fears control the way they live, they decide to get on with life in spite of their fears.

Here are some ways of dealing with worries that pop into your head and cause you to feel fearful:

What if I start a weight loss programme and I fail?
Every time a worrying 'what if' pops into your head, you are more than likely going to experience fear and this will lead to in-decisiveness and powerlessness. So it's important that you replace the 'what if' statement with a 'so what' statement.

So what if I start a weight loss programme and I fail.
You will feel less afraid if you look at the challenges ahead in the light of 'so what' instead of 'what if'. As you proceed with your weight loss and worrying, self-defeating thoughts return to nag you, always ask yourself:
What is the worst thing that could happen?

This will help you put things in perspective and not regard the least little hiccup as a complete catastrophe! Picture the fol-lowing scenario:

You have lost a stone and you start worrying that you are not going to keep to your plan and you'll put it all back on again. You think in terms of 'what if' and you tell yourself you are going to feel such a failure, people will talk about you, you will be ashamed, and so on. But so what if your weight loss plans go awry, what really is the worst thing that could happen? You will go back to living the way you are now but remember, it will be different because you will have learned from your experience of failing and you will be armed with new knowledge which will enable you to look at new options.

For example, if you failed to lose weight last time because the diet you followed denied you the foods you loved and in the end you simply could not stick it any longer, next time you know you need to follow a balanced diet that allows you more leeway. You can either punish yourself after a relapse from your healthy eating plan or use it as an opportunity to learn and recognise pitfalls earlier next time.

Questions to ask yourself:
√ With this relapse what can I learn?
√ Why am I holding onto my weight?
√ Is there any gain?

What we sometimes forget when we face new challenges is that we have succeeded in many ways in our lives. In our anxious moments, we overlook our successes and exaggerate our failures.

In your notebook, list your past successes and give yourself credit for them. If you succeeded before, there's no reason why you can't do so again. Now list the times you have failed in the past and ask yourself if these experiences were really a waste of time. What are the positive things you can learn from them? So often we allow our failures to haunt us and keep us stuck in the weight trap. What we need to do is learn from the times we have failed to lose weight, put it down to experience and move on. Anything that stops you from losing weight is reinforcing a negative self-limiting belief that you cannot change.

Keep the following in mind when your fear of failing stops you from achieving your weight loss dream:

- It's okay to feel afraid, it doesn't mean I have to give up. I can still feel this way and continue my healthy eating plan.
- I will not let my fears control the way I live. I will become aware of them and learn from them to create something new and exciting in my life.
- I don't identify with my fears or criticise myself because of them. My fears do not define who I am.
- I will not let my fears make me postpone my weight loss plans.

Please note: It is important to seek professional help if fear and anxiety are interfering with your life on an ongoing basis.

Homework: Create your own life chart

All the tasks in this book are like pieces of a jigsaw – as each piece fits into place, you are creating a *new you* who is conquering a weight problem and living a healthier and happier life.

Before progressing to the next chapter, fill out the *life chart* that follows. This chart asks you to recall your good and bad memories at different ages. Try to remember what weight you were with each memory you write. An example of what people generally write in this chart is also included (see p. 49).

In creating your own *life chart*, you are becoming aware of how your circumstances influence your weight. If you are now a busy working mum, for example, you may be feeling very stressed and start overeating because of it. Or maybe you have retired, are not as active as you used to be and you are becoming overweight. By charting your good and bad memories, you will be further developing the *getting to know you* process and understanding why you are overweight now.

Life Chart Example

AGE	GOOD MEMORIES	BAD MEMORIES
0–5	Loving family occasions, holidays, starting school.	Feeling bigger than other children, having difficulties making friends.
6–11	Achievements at school and in art and drama.	Starting to put on more weight. Premature development, being bullied because of weight.
12–19	Happy time in school, learn horse riding.	Yo-yo dieting, hating myself, depression.
20-29	Graduated from college.	Not getting job I wanted because of weight, hating holidays because of feeling fat, struggling and being hurt in relationships.
30–45	Loving relationship, becoming a parent, success at work.	Putting on weight, having children and letting the weight continue to pile on as the years pass.
46–59	Paying off the mortgage, taking things a little easier at work, having more time to spend with family and friends.	Children aren't turning out the way I expected, struggling with growing old, unhappy with how I look and finding comfort in food.
60+	Weddings of children, grandchildren born.	Retired with too much time on my hands, spouse ill/dies, feeling lonely and overeating to escape the pain.

My life chart

AGE	GOOD MEMORIES	BAD MEMORIES
0–5		
6–11		
12–19		
20–29		
30–45		
46–59		
60+		

DOs and DON'Ts for life chart

• Do be realistic. Your memories may not be a true reflection of everything that happened, so don't regard them as facts. Instead, use your *life chart* to understand how much the good and bad things that happen to us influence the way we think, feel and behave.

• Don't dwell on the bad memories. The purpose of this chart is to help you get to know who you are and how you got to where you are today. Remember to look at your good memories as well.

- Do give yourself credit for all the good things you have achieved in life.
- Don't blame yourself for things over which you had no control. Instead, use today as the start of a new time in your life.
- Do seek professional help if there are issues you need to deal with. Remember your general practitioner is always your first port of call.

6

Riding Life's Roller Coaster

Life is full of surprises. When we get up in the morning, we just don't know what the day will bring. While we can have certain plans in place – going to work, going shopping, meeting friends for lunch – none of us can predict what we will do precisely, or what will happen in the hours that follow. It's inevitable that events occur every day which are beyond our control, sometimes they bring happiness and joy (a long lost friend phones up out of the blue), other times stress and anxiety (you find out you are being made redundant). How we react to events outside our control determines how successful we are at maintaining a sense of inner peace and happiness during the highs and the lows of life.

We suggest that you develop a coping strategy so that you are prepared for these events and can avoid destructive reactions such as overeating. We call this your *resource management strategy*. When we use the word 'resources', we often think of assets such as money and possessions, but resources also include our attributes, skills, energy, time, confidence, support mechanisms and personal relationships. You will have many of these resources already, others you may need to develop.

RESOURCE 1: PERSONAL OUTLOOK

Self-Acceptance
Being slim does not make you superior as a human being, and conversely being overweight does not make you inferior. We have stated already in this book that we are all fallible beings with a variety of strengths and weakness. While we are happy with our strengths, we do not look badly upon ourselves because

of our weaknesses. Rather we develop a healthy self-acceptance of them. In other words, we accept that we don't do so well in some areas of our lives and we always strive to change and improve. Without self-acceptance you may find it difficult to escape from the weight trap. Telling yourself you are overweight and useless will not get you anywhere, so learn to love yourself warts and all.

Self-confidence

In Chapter 2, we showed you how to improve your confidence by changing the way you think. In the last chapter, we pointed out that conquering your fears is about being willing to take the chance that you will succeed and then simply just going for it! Confidence often comes as a result of doing something, not before. If you are waiting to feel confident before you lose weight, you could be waiting a long time. This doesn't mean that you have no inner confidence, it just takes a small achievement on your road to weight loss to feel more confident. As you draw nearer your goal and your achievements mount up, your confidence also improves.

Approach to self and the world

Often we are our own worst enemies. We criticise ourselves far more than we need to and end up with low self-esteem. A healthy attitude to ourselves – one that is realistic and accepts that we are not perfect – is reflected in the way we relate to other people and how we react to events. If our expectations are unrealistic, we will not be happy with ourselves or anyone else. A rigid, perfectionist outlook makes living difficult, so our motto is: Always be gentle with yourself.

Resource 2: Life Skills

We all have a variety of skills and if we are asked to consider them in terms of our jobs, they trip off our tongues. However, we tend to overlook many of our other life skills, which are extremely important in helping us create balance in our lives. We have categorised such skills under the headings of Personal Management, Relationship, Outlook, and Self-Care. See if you can identify with some or all of them and see which ones you would like to develop.

Personal Management Skills:

Valuing: investing in myself
Planning: moving towards my goal
Commitment: saying yes
Time use: setting priorities
Pacing: controlling the tempo

Relationship Skills:

Contact: reaching out to others
Listening: tuning into others
Assertiveness: saying no
Fight: standing your ground
Flight: leaving the scene
Nest building: creating a health positive home

Outlook Skills:

Re-labelling: a new perspective
Surrender: saying 'goodbye'
Faith: accepting your limits
Imagination: laughing, creating
Whisper: talking nicely to yourself

Self-Care Skills:

Exercise: fine-tuning the body
Eating: feeding healthy food
Gentleness: wearing kid gloves
Relaxation: letting go of tension
Stretching: loosening up

Now consider the following – at the present moment:

What are your best skills?

What are your undeveloped skills?

Which skills do you use most often?

Which are your under-utilised skills?

Identify the skills important to your future weight loss:

Skills I've neglected – I'd like to use again.

Skills I'm no good at, but I'd like to learn and practise.

Skills I'd like to maintain and I'll need.

Skills I'd like to use less and put on the back burner for now.

By honing our skills, we are taking another important step on our journey of self-change and weight loss.

RESOURCE 3: OTHER PEOPLE

Research has shown that good social support helps improve our immune function and recovery prospects in any illness. Comfort eaters frequently report retreating from relationships and activities because they feel inadequate. Sometimes family tend not to ask how a weight loss programme is going for fear of not knowing how to help. Positive support groups have been clinically shown to improve prognosis. Remember, however, some people find one-to-one support better, so choose what works best for you. Communicate with your family and tell them how they can help you. If you are seeking professional support, you will find a list of contact organisations on pages 122 and 123.

If you haven't the courage now to ask for help, in a later chapter we will show you how to make that important step.

Homework: Create your own self-management plan

The unconscious mind effectively manages our body and we achieve more each day if we have well-defined targets and outcomes. People addressing a weight problem are often experiencing significant degrees of confusion in thinking. In order to stay focused on your weight loss goal, it's a good idea to equip yourself with a *self-management plan* that leads you to clearer outcomes.

Take your time answering the questions. There are no right or wrong answers. Your answers, if you are really honest with yourself, will help enhance the clarity of your unconscious mind and help slow down the roller coaster of emotions and thoughts that are leading to distorted thinking and overeating.

In your notebook, answer the following questions:

1   What do you want from your weight loss programme (not what you don't want)?
2   What are you already doing to achieve your weight loss?
3   What stage are you at now? This is a good time to assess your progress.
4   What will you continue to do to achieve your outcome?
5   What will achieving your target weight do for you?
6   Who will benefit the most?
7   How specifically will your family benefit?
8   How will you know when you have achieved your outcome?
9   What stops you now or might stop you in the future from reaching your goal?
10   Are there any additional resources or support mechanisms that you might need, and what are they?
11   At what stage would it be beneficial to have additional resources in place?
12   How will you benefit from achieving help/support from additional resources?
13   What will you lose by achieving your goal?
14   How worthwhile is that goal for you to persist with the process of change?

☞ Tools for action

You have come to end of Step 3 on your journey to weight loss and you are now ready to take *the gamble that you will succeed.*

Here is a reminder of your *tools for action* before you progress to the next step.

- If fear of failure is immobilising you, it's time to think seriously if you want to live this way the rest of your life.
- Use the language of 'so what' instead of 'what if' and turn your fear into something positive.
- Even if you do not succeed, you will learn from the experience of failing. Let your motto be: If at first I don't succeed, I will try, try again.
- You do not need to use food as a crutch during bad times. Develop a *resource management strategy* which helps you draw on all your inner strengths as well as on the support of family, loved ones, friends and professional help.
- In order to be clear about why you want to lose weight and what you hope to achieve, draw up a *self-management plan.*
- Always bear in mind that there are many peaks and valleys on the road to weight loss, so be realistic and don't expect to get everything right all of the time. We are all works in progress after all!

I used to try every fad diet and think that I could lose weight instantly. Once, I lost a stone in a fortnight and put it back on in a month. When I reached my goal, I couldn't stay there.

STEP 4

ONLY SET GOALS YOU CAN ACHIEVE

7

Getting to Where You Want to Be

There once was a man who waited all his life to be happy. The last anyone heard of him, he was still waiting.

ROBERT HOLDEN

One of the main obstacles to achieving goals is procrastination, putting things on the long finger. As we've pointed out before, in-action is often caused by fear of failure, but if you wonder how other people achieve their weight loss goal, it's simply because one day they decided to give it a try. If you wait until you feel really motivated you could be waiting forever, so whether you feel like it or not, take action now!

Motivation can be the difference between someone who transforms their life and someone who languishes in a boring but comfortable rut. If you are motivated, you can really do almost anything with your life, from revitalising a relationship to taking on a new career, or losing weight. So, if you find it hard to get motivated, here is how to do it:

1. Get Started

Get started on your weight loss plan and as you see results, you will feel more confident and motivated. Then it will be easier to keep going. Dr Moore-Groarke often says to patients: 'procrastination is your greatest sin, don't put things off, do it now'. If you can avoid putting things on the long finger, face your fears and act now, you will be setting yourself up for success. Once you tackle your weight problems, everything else will seem a lot easier.

2. Be Realistic

Remember that having unrealistic expectations leads to disappointment, so be realistic and expect that some weeks you may not lose any weight. Break your goals down into small achievable milestones. For every milestone reached, give yourself credit and treat yourself to something nice (see *treats ideas* in this chapter). Remain positive throughout and use a healthy weight loss and exercise programme together with the tools you have learned in this book to get to goal and stay there.

3. Get in Control

It isn't easy to change everything at once. Make a treasure map with images of the things you want to achieve in your life. Put a picture of yourself in the middle and under it, write the word 'control'. This map will talk directly to your subconscious and is a marvellous way of subtly motivating yourself.

4. Clear Out the Clutter

Clear out the clutter at home and work because clutter muddles the mind and can keep us stuck in the past. Forget about dwelling on the past because it is a total de-motivator. Know where everything is, what foods are in the fridge, and so on. Clarity of mind comes after such a spring clean.

5. Surround Yourself with Positive People

Joan Collins is a great believer in only keeping positive people around her. Attend a weight loss class with a positive leader who will motivate you towards weight loss. Let a supportive friend, who is not trying to compete with you, encourage you to take exercise. Enlist the help of your partner and family so that they can inspire you, but remember to *always take responsibility for your own actions*. Seek the support of others but don't base your success on their approval of you. Lose weight for you and you alone.

6. Choose Creative Challenges

Creativity is another important key to change and to increased motivation. Try out new things; meet new people. Each week choose a small new challenge for yourself and achieving it will be a great self-esteem and confidence booster.

7. Manage Your Time

Have some time each day to relax so that this 'You Time' will aid control regarding healthy eating. While it may seem obsessive at the outset, use your diary to slot in each activity you need to complete on a daily basis. Don't over commit and burn yourself out. Postpone something by prioritising the activities that help you to learn to take control. Later, we give pointers for avoiding stress.

8. Manage Your Moods

If you are in a bad mood, it's a lot easier to overeat. It is important to programme our brains by starting and finishing each day doing something that generates a physical feeling of well being and relaxation. Later, we help you discover ways you can achieve a healthy life balance.

Please note: if you are regularly prone to mood swings you may be suffering from depression and may need to consult your doctor for advice.

Rules for goal-setting

When setting goals, the golden rule is that we are realistic about what we can achieve, that way our desires won't lead to disappointment and disillusionment. If, for example, we want to get fit and we haven't been involved in any formal exercise since we left school, we will need to start gradually and build up our stamina levels over time. Expecting to be an Olympic athlete in a month would just not be realistic!

In order to reach our goals, we need to:

- Be aware of the changes we need to make.
- Develop a realistic plan of action.
- Break our target goal into smaller achievable goals.
- Learn from the times when we lapse and remain focused on our goal.
- Give ourselves credit when we achieve our goal.

TREAT YOURSELF – YOU DESERVE IT!

Losing weight is not about punishing yourself but about loving yourself more. So make sure you give yourself credit for all you achieve along the way (no matter how small the milestone), and take every opportunity to treat yourself. If you really feel like a food treat, opt for a low-fat alternative but whenever possible, choose a non-food treat *instead because there will be no danger of regressive eating patterns. Here are some non-food treat ideas:*

A Short Holiday
If you feel a little tired, a break away can work wonders for the mind and body. The joy of having your bed made and your breakfast cooked is such a treat, as is getting away from the usual day-to-day chores. You can also use this short break to avail of healthy exercise activities in the area – swimming, walking, cycling, surfing, or whatever else takes your fancy! One thing is sure – if you make the most of the break, you will return home refreshed and rejuvenated.

A Beauty Treatment
There are lots of beauty treatments available these days, from standard grooming such as manicures and pedicures to alternative spa treatments that include massage and other relaxation methods. Taking time out to take care of your body is an important way of finding a space where you can wind down and let our worries waft away. By learning to relax, you will both look and feel better.

A Bubbly Bath
It may not be possible to go for beauty treatments every week but hav-

ing a long, warm soak in the bath is something we can do anytime. Create a relaxing atmosphere in your bathroom by dimming the lights or lighting some aromatherapy candles or incense. Run a warm bath and use your favourite beauty products to wash your body, doing everything at a slow, gentle pace. Have soft, warm towels ready for afterwards and you will feel really pampered and relaxed.

A Relaxation Class

Some people find it more difficult than others do to relax. If you have high energy levels and you're usually running around the place, then it can be hard to slow down. Making a weekly appointment to go to a relaxation class is one way of disciplining yourself to take time out. At a class such as yoga or t'ai chi, you will learn methods of relaxation that you can then practise at home. The other advantage of going out to a class is that it's a great way to meet new people and forget about your own cares.

A Shopping Trip

Make a date with yourself, or better still hook up with a friend, to go shopping at least once a month and as you lose weight, you will discover that you enjoy shopping all the more. Fitting into a trendy new outfit is a great way of reminding yourself of how far you have come and what you have achieved.

Buy a Book/Go to the Cinema

If you enjoy reading, treat yourself to a new book and take time out to read it and enjoy it every day. Or perhaps you love the cinema but haven't been there in ages – do whatever it takes to get to see a movie even if it means booking a babysitter.

Symbol of change

We suggest you buy a symbol of change, for example a poster, fridge magnet, or soft toy, something that you will see each day and represents the *new you*, what you hope to achieve with your weight loss plan.

Another idea is to buy a packet of flower seeds and sow them, either in your garden or in a plant pot. As you move towards your goal, the seeds you have sown will also be growing and developing, eventually turning into colourful flowers, and will represent a very real symbol of change for you and your new life.

Homework: Create a goal hierarchy
Set out a goal hierarchy over the next six months and in doing so, remember to be realistic. Each level on the hierarchy represents one month. As you move up the levels, the goals become a little harder. Six-month hierarchies are a realistic time frame in which to review your progress.

Below is an example of such a hierarchy based on a target of one stone weight loss.

HIERARCHY OF GOALS FOR WEIGHT LOSS

Levels	*Goals*	*Months*
Level 6	*1 stone weight loss: reward of a weekend away*	⭕ Month 6 ◉
Level 5	*Give up cigarettes. Continue healthy eating and exercise pattern. Seek support at my weight loss class.*	⭕ Month 5 ◉
Level 4	*Learn to cook interesting healthy meals. Leave the car at home 1 day a week. Continue attending my weight loss class.*	⭕ Month 4 ◉
Level 3	*Adopt a daily exercise routine combined with relaxation. Half stone weight loss and look good for a special event.*	⭕ Month 3 ◉
Level 2	*Educate myself more about healthy eating. Plan exercise for the month ahead. Seek advice at my weight loss class.*	⭕ Month 2 ◉
Level 1	*Join a weight loss class. Slow down when I am eating. Learn to relax. Make out a shopping list.*	⭕ Month 1 ◉

HOMEWORK: MY HIERARCHY OF GOALS

Levels	Goals	Months
Level 6		
Level 5		
Level 4		
Level 3		
Level 2		
Level 1		

8

Daring to Imagine

Willpower is a conscious process where we use choice positively and completely. We often talk about people who have great willpower. They have managed to give up cigarettes, stay off the booze, stop biting their nails, triumph over a gambling addiction, and so on. We admire them and wonder why we can't do the same when it comes to food. There is one simple answer to this: it is much more difficult to tackle behaviour around food. We must eat to live and therefore we can never avoid eating. While the alcoholic can avoid going into a pub and avoid alcohol most of the time, somebody who is on a diet can never avoid food. Therefore, it is much more difficult to rely on our willpower alone. That's why we need to support our willpower by tapping into our creative side and drawing on the power of our imagination to sustain us in the long-term.

Ask yourself the following:

√ How committed are you to losing weight?
√ Are you willing to persist with changing your lifestyle?
√ Do you understand that healthy eating is both a physical and
   psychological process?

If you answer 'Yes' to all of these questions, then you are ready to use your imagination to help you stick with your healthy eating programme.

Imagine how you wish your body to be. This is the reality you can create.

Research has shown that a relaxed person will achieve greater weight loss, and over the years, Dr Moore-Groarke has found that people struggling with food cravings benefit from creating a relaxation script that they put on audiotape. The following is an example of a relaxation script you can put on tape yourself. We recommend using the tape at least once a day or, if you have the time to spare, every morning and every evening. Practising relaxation techniques every day is far more effective than only using them when we feel the urge to overeat or eat for the sake of it.

The purpose of this tape is to practise deep relaxation, to relax so deeply that every time you think of eating when you're not hungry, or overeating, these thoughts disappear. Using this technique, you can get into a relaxed frame of mind and thoughts of leading a healthy life sink down deep into your subconscious where they can have maximum effect.

Homework: Create a relaxation tape
Record the following *introduction* and *now it's time to relax* on an audiotape. If you don't like listening to your own voice on tape, ask a friend or family member who has a soothing voice to make the tape for you.

Introduction
As you listen to this introduction, get into a relaxed position ...

Food is a necessary ingredient in life for all of us, part of our daily routine but also part of most celebrations. Food is one of life's pleasures. But some of us don't enjoy food because we don't use it responsibly. We mistreat the wonderful gift that food is by overeating and putting our health at risk.

On this tape you will hear a demonstration of deep muscle relaxation and how you can make yourself so relaxed that every time you have thoughts of eating too much or using food irresponsibly, these thoughts will disappear. You can learn to relax so deeply that you can rid yourself of all tension and nervousness around food, you can learn to choose where food is concerned – choose to eat healthily, choose to escape from the weight trap, choose to really enjoy food.

This form of relaxation is recommended by the medical profession, it is now commonly used in the treatment of many conditions. When you learn to relax, your thoughts become more positive, you recognise clearly the need to change your behaviour, you have a better chance at leading a normal life, and you can learn to regain your confidence.

Now just for one moment, think of all the ways you can benefit if you learn to relax and face up to your weight problem. Think of your weight problem and then without any strain, think of what it would be like if you where free from this problem. Consistently and consciously day after day, you will make time to allow your thoughts to sink into your mind so that you will learn to be in control. You can choose not to allow food to control your life.

When you learn deep muscle relaxation, you should find that you can sit down alone any time during the day and practise this relaxation. The reasons why food controls you will become more apparent and in time, once you work through these issues, you can learn to accept and love yourself again. All negative thoughts and behaviour will disappear.

Now it's time to relax …
Close your eyes and make sure you are in the most relaxed position you can find … Become aware of your thoughts of food and allow them one by one to drift away … As you concentrate on a sense of relaxation, you will notice the tension and nervousness disappear … As your muscles feel at ease, your body will become warm and heavy but deeply relaxed … Become aware of how good your body feels and stay in this position for about ten seconds …

Now focus on each part of your body … Concentrate first on

your left leg ... Focus your attention on each part of your leg in turn ... Starting with your toes and working towards your hip ... As you work up your leg, feel the tension drift away ... Notice the sensation of warmth, limpness and heaviness relax your toes ... Count to five (in your head) ... Relax the instep ... Count to five ... Relax the heel ... Count to five ... Relax the ankle ... Count to five ... Relax the calf muscles ... Count to five ... Feel how warm, limp and heavy the calf muscles become ... Relax the knee ... Count to five ... Relax the thigh ... Count to five ... Relax your hip ... Count to five ... Concentrate on this wonderful feeling of relaxation in your left leg ... Count to five ... Warm, limp, and heavy ... Your thoughts of food are drifting away ...

Now focus your attention on your right leg, paying attention to each part of your leg in turn, starting with your toes and working towards your hip ... As you work up your leg, feel the tension drift away, notice the sensation of warmth, limpness, and heaviness ... Relax your toes ... Count to five ... Relax the instep ... Count to five ... The heel ... Count to five ... The ankle ... Count to five ... Relax the calf muscles ... Count to five, feel how warm and heavy they become ... Relax the knee ... Count to five ... The thigh ... Count to five ... And your hips ... Count to five ... Concentrate on this wonderful feeling of relaxation in your right leg ... Count to five, warm, limp, and heavy ... Your thoughts of food are drifting away ...

Now concentrate on your left arm ... Focus your attention on each part of your left arm in turn, starting with your fingers and working towards your shoulder ... Relax your fingers and thumb ... Count to five ... Feel them curl inwards ... Count to five ... Relax your palm ... Count to five ... Now your wrist ... Count to five ... Your forearm ... Count to five ... Your elbow ... Count to five ... Your upper arm ... Count to five ... And lastly, your shoulder ... Count to five, concentrate on the warm, limp and heavy sensation ... Your thoughts of food are drifting away ...

Now concentrate on your right arm ... Focus your attention

on each part of your right arm in turn, starting with your fingers and working towards your shoulder ... Relax your fingers and thumb ... Count to five ... Feel them curl inwards ... Count to five ... Relax your palm ... Count to five ... Now your wrist ... Count to five ... Your forearm ... Count to five ... Your elbow ... Count to five ... Your upper arm ... Count to five ... And lastly, your shoulder ... Count to five, concentrate on the warm, limp and heavy sensation ... Your thoughts of food are drifting away ...

Now focus on your stomach muscles, notice how your stomach feels when you learn to relax it ... You can learn to see it as it really is, not how you imagine it to be ... Relax your stomach ... Count to five ...

Now concentrate on the base of your spine, slowly work your way up your spine towards the neck, relaxing each bone of the spine and the muscles around it ... As you progress towards the neck, feel the muscles relax, becoming warm, limp and heavy as your back sinks into a relaxed position ...

As you are learning how good it feels to relax, you are re-cognising you have choice where food is concerned ...

Now relax your shoulders ... Count to five ... Feel them drop towards the floor ... Count to five ... They are warm, heavy and limp... Your thoughts of food are drifting away ...

Now relax your neck muscles, keep your head straight, your spine parallel to the floor ... Your head is now balanced on your spine ...

You will learn how not to let food rule your life ...

Now focus your attention on your head ... Relax your jaw ... Count to five ... Let it drop to your mouth ... Feel your mouth slightly open ... Count to five ... Relax your tongue ... Count to five ... And feel it drop behind your lower teeth ... Count to five ... Relax the muscles around your eyes ... Count to five ... Feel them become warm, limp and heavy ... Count to five ... Your scalp ... Count to five ...

Your head should be totally relaxed warm and heavy, your

thoughts of food have disappeared ...

Become aware of your breathing ... Feel your abdominal muscles move out and up as you inhale and exhale slowly and gently ... Breathe in and out ... in and out ... Notice how good this feels ... Now relax, count to five ...

Quieten you mind, allow all your thoughts drift away, drift away through your heart without trying to pursue them ... As easily as your thoughts reappear you can allow them to disappear ... You are in control as you can be in control of your food ...

Picture yourself walking along the seashore ... It's your beach and the waves are lapping up and down ... Feel your feet sink deep into the sand ... It's warm and you are deeply relaxed ... The sky is a deep blue and cloudless ... You become aware of the sounds around you ... You are deeply relaxed ... You are in control ...

Stay quietly in this position for about five minutes and enjoy this wonderful state of relaxation that you have created throughout your body ... You feel good, relaxed and totally in control ... Your body feels warm and heavy ... You are so relaxed that you can now face the world ... Food has become less of a problem ...

When you open your eyes will feel refreshed and relaxed and find that you have the choice to learn to change your behaviour and live a normal life again.

☞ *Tools for action*
You have come to the end of Step 4 where we have encouraged you to *only set goals you can achieve*.

There has been quite a lot to do in this chapter, so here is reminder:

√ Stop putting your weight loss on the long finger. Take action now, not tomorrow or next Monday morning.

√ Set realistic, achievable goals. Draw up a hierarchy of goals over a 6-month period. Tackle the easier goals in the first month.

√ Have realistic expectations of what is achievable and give yourself credit for your successes.

√ Treat yourself along the way to non-food treats. You deserve it!

√ Use the power of your imagination to practice deep relaxation to strengthen your resolve and help your escape from the weight trap.

I have great intentions to eat healthily but when I feel stressed, I just have to eat lots of sugary things. It's the only way I can keep going.

STEP 5

BECOME AWARE OF YOUR TRIGGERS

9

Finding Out if You are Really Hungry

Eating is a pleasurable experience and therefore we often eat when not hungry. Have you ever wondered why you eat a bar of chocolate when you are watching your favourite TV programme? Why you like eating popcorn at the cinema? Why you overeat when you feel emotionally vulnerable – maybe lonely, anxious, depressed?

When considering our behaviour around food, it is important to ask: *Am I physically hungry?* or *Am I psychologically hungry?*

When you eat according to physical hunger, you use the thinking side of your brain. You understand that you only need to eat a certain amount to survive and stay healthy. Your healthy eating programme has educated you about following a balanced diet, you understand this and are able to put it into action. You respect and appreciate food and you know that if you overeat, it will no longer be enjoyable.

The emotional side of your brain governs psychological hunger. When you eat according to psychological hunger, you use foods to anaesthetise your feelings. Much of your psychological hunger is learned behaviour habits, such as eating sweets when you cried as a child. You need to try to unlearn these behaviours and confront the belief that food can be used as a substitute for something else other than hunger. A patient of Dr Moore-Groarke once commented: 'The only way my mother was ever able to show me love was by feeding me.' This patient went on to develop eating problems later in life.

If you cut your knee, would you put a plaster on it? For people in emotional pain, that plaster may be food. This is when your eating habits are controlling you and keeping you stuck in the weight trap. Food does not solve emotional problems – you may feel temporary escape but a continuous cycle of overeating, as we have pointed out in Step 1, will lead to low self-esteem and general feelings of worthlessness.

Identifying your triggers

Once you have established whether it is physical or psychological hunger that is causing you to overeat, the next step is developing a strategy to make healthy choices. The first thing we want you to do is look over your diaries and notes from previous chapters to help you identify what causes you to overeat. We all have different triggers, such as watching TV, loneliness, shopping, boredom, low self-esteem, bad habits, and so on.

Triggers can be divided into the following categories. Become aware of what triggers you to overeat and develop an action plan by making good everyday decisions. Remember it is the small changes we make to our eating habits that can determine success or failure in the long-term.

	Yes	No
Emotional Triggers		
Do you overeat when you are bored, lonely, depressed?	☐	☐
Sight Triggers		
Do you decide to eat just because you see somebody else eating?	☐	☐
Smell Triggers		
Does the smell of cooking food tempt you to eat?	☐	☐
Association Triggers		
Do you associate an experience with eating e.g., watching television?	☐	☐
Subliminal Triggers		
Do you eat certain foods because the advertisement appeals to you?	☐	☐

Decide how you might tackle psychological hunger, for example write down what is going through your mind – instead of giving in to the food, ring a friend and have a chat, go for a walk, do something not related to food. Practice will make perfect. Once you overcome the initial craving, you will feel stronger.

See the *triggers table* below for some ideas. We have included situations where we feel physical hunger and where we feel psychological hunger – for both situations we need to make healthy choices in order to develop healthy eating habits that will ensure long-term weight loss.

TRIGGERS TABLE EXAMPLE

Time	Situation	Feelings Before Food
11am	Coffee break at work	Hungry
4pm	At home alone with baby	Lonely
6pm	Arrive home from work	Hungry
8pm	Get a call to say I didn't get the job I want	Rejected and worthless
8.30pm	At home, thinking about presentation I have to make at work tomorrow	Anxious
9pm	At the cinema, smell popcorn	'Peckish'
9.30pm	At the restaurant with friends	Happy

For those peckish times

In the *triggers table*, we listed the feeling of 'peckishness'. When we feel peckish, we may think we are physically hungry but, in reality, we are psychologically hungry. In other words, we think we are hungry but in fact we are not hungry at all! These can be the trickiest situations when it comes to your weight loss plan – if you avoid eating every time you are peckish you may end up feeling deprived and find your diet boring.

That's why it's a good idea to have a balanced diet that includes eating healthy foods and taking exercise, but still gives you

Thoughts Before Food	Unhealthy Response	Healthy Response
I had no breakfast. I need to eat	Tuck into a scone with full fat butter	Have a slice of bread with low-fat spread
I have no friends. I'm fed up	Eat chocolate and a packet of crisps	Go for a walk with baby
I am so hungry I cannot wait to cook dinner	Have a cup of tea and three slices of bread with jam before I cook dinner	Have an apple and then cook dinner
I am a loser I will never get a job	Order a pizza delivery with garlic bread and lie on the couch watching television	Eat a low fat meal and call a friend for a chat
I will make a mess of the presentation	Make a cup of tea and eat a slice of cream cake	Have a relaxing bath and listen to some music
The smell of popcorn is delicious	Buy a large container of popcorn	Opt for low fat, no-butter popcorn in smaller container
I love being with friends. I feel wonderful	Throw caution to the wind and have a meal with all the works	Have a meal with two courses – either skip the starter or the dessert

some leeway to indulge a little occasionally. A sensible weight loss programme will help you get that balance right. Most of the time, however, it's wise to have low-fat alternatives or non-food treats lined up for the times we feel peckish.

Here is a list of situations in which many people feel peckish. Tick the ones that apply to you:

Watching TV in the evening	☐
At the cinema	☐
Having tea/coffee	☐
Mid-afternoon after a heavy lunch	☐
Shopping in the supermarket	☐
Sitting around with nothing to do	☐
Driving in the car	☐
Going on a bus or train journey	☐
Before bedtime	☐

To explain further, let's look at one of these situations in more detail – shopping at the supermarket. Picture the following scenarios:

√ You have finished work and you are doing the week's shopping. You've had a hard day and you're feeling really tired and hungry. You hadn't planned to buy any chocolate but while waiting at the cash register, you reach out and put a bar into your basket. As you pack your groceries in the car, your tummy is rumbling and you decide to tuck into the bar of chocolate on the way home.

√ You have had a main meal and now you are in the supermarket shopping for a light, healthy meal for your tea. However, your plans go awry once you smell chickens cooking at the deli counter. Although you hadn't planned to buy a cooked chicken, the aroma is making you feel hungry and you buy it on impulse. When you arrive home, you eat far more than you had planned.

√ You have planned this week to limit the amount of biscuits and cakes you buy, the theory being, if they aren't in your cupboard it will be more difficult to eat them. However, when shopping at the local supermarket you discover that there's a special offer this week on your favourite biscuits. You can buy three packs for the price of one. It's a fantastic bargain and you just can't resist it! As a result, you eat three times as many biscuits this week as you had planned.

As you can see from the above scenarios, many things trigger us to overeat. As well as our own feelings of physical hunger and tiredness, other factors come into play such as the aroma of the cooked chickens and the bargain offers.

Tips for supermarket shopping
Here are some tips to help you shop wisely. You can create your own strategy for other ways you are triggered to overeat.

√ Make out a shopping list in advance and stick to it.
√ Try not to shop when you're hungry because you might be tempted to buy more than you need.
√ Read labels carefully. If something is 5% fat free, remember it has a fat content of 95%.
√ Look out for low-fat alternatives to the foods you normally buy.
√ Don't be tempted to buy in bulk just because of supermarket bargains. Keep your shopping list in mind!
√ If you feel peckish on your way home from shopping, have a low-fat snack such as a piece of fruit or a low calorie cereal bar.

Tips for breaking bad habits
Our eating habits can be changed if we so choose. Repeating the process of change leads to adaption. It takes at least twenty repetitions for a habit to be formed so, in order to break bad habits, be prepared to put in a lot of effort at the beginning. If you are in the habit of having biscuits with tea, for example, decide to break

this habit by having nothing with your cup of tea for a while. Then, every so often, you can choose to have a biscuit with your tea and enjoy it. Here are some other choices you can make:

1 Eat at regular times and follow a diet that nourishes your body with lots of vitamins and minerals. That way you will feel less tired and will not crave high sugar foods as much.
2 Eat your meals in a civilised fashion, sit at the table and eat with a knife and fork. Savour and enjoy every mouthful and you will be giving your brain the chance to know that you are feeling full. It takes a little while for our brains to register that our physical hunger has been satisfied, therefore if you eat in a hurry, you will have eaten too much before you begin to realise you are full. Always leave the table feeling you could eat a little more.
3 Give your taste buds a chance to change. You may not love the taste of vegetables at first but if you persist in eating them on a daily basis, you will soon always want vegetables with your main meal.
4 Do not skip a meal or you may be tempted to keep your energy levels up by picking at fatty foods. When your energy levels are low or you are feeling peckish, opt for low-fat alternatives such as fresh fruit. Keep a bowl of fruit stocked up, have low fat alternatives in your fridge/cupboard, at work, in your car – situations where you may get peckish between meals.
5 Be flexible in your weight loss plan and allow yourself occasional food treats because if you feel deprived, you will not be able to maintain this plan for the rest of your life. It's a good idea to limit the quantities of treats, for example choose to have two pieces of chocolate instead of six.
6 Reward yourself regularly with non-food treats such as going for a walk, having a bath, listening to music, going to the hairdresser, and so on.

7 If you crave food, do not give in immediately. Book a time with yourself – saying in an hour or two, I will have two pieces of chocolate. This way you limit the destruction.

8 Be imaginative in your cooking and put colour and variety into your diet. This way you will find healthy eating interesting and pleasurable.

9 If your social life revolves around food, start enjoying time in people's company by doing something different. For example, if you regularly meet friends for coffee and cake, meet them for a walk instead, or meet them at meal times rather than in between meals.

10 Take responsibility for your own eating behaviour. Nobody can make you overeat – only you! Excuses are no substitute for willpower. Sometimes, it can be difficult to keep to your healthy eating plan, especially if something such as the smell of food triggers you to eat. Become aware of your triggers and stay focused on your weight loss goal.

Assessing your food fears

In a previous chapter, we discussed fear in the context of holding us back from our weight loss dreams. Fear can also play a significant role in dictating how and where we eat. For example, when alone we often eat differently than in company. Sometimes the fear of what other people think of us forces us to make so-called healthy choices in front of them. Or for example, if you are trying to follow a weight loss plan, you can also be fearful of your triggers. By having a strategy for these fearful situations in place, however, there is no need to be afraid. The best strategy involves facing up to your fears in a gentle, gradual manner. Always remember if you do lapse, you can pick yourself up and start again.

FOOD FEARS TABLE EXAMPLE

By becoming aware of our food fears, we can assess which ones are the greatest, and start putting a strategy in place to conquer them.

Situation	Strength of Fear 0–20%	Strength of Fear 21–40%	Strength of Fear 41–70%	Strength of Fear 71–100%
In the company of colleagues				
In a restaurant looking at menu				
Smelling food and unable to resist it				
Family member prepares a high fat meal for you				
Eating with somebody who is slim				

Homework: Create your own triggers table

Earlier we created an example of a *triggers table* in which we showed how we eat according to physical and psychological hunger. We suggest that for one week, you record what you eat and when you eat during the day in the *triggers table* below (you will need to make extra copies for your self). This table will help you become aware of the situations, feelings and thoughts which trigger you to overeat. Your response to these triggers can be healthy or unhealthy. These everyday choices will be the difference between being slim for life or having to cope with being overweight and all that it entails.

MY TRIGGERS TABLE
Day 1

Time	Situation	Feelings Before Food	Thoughts Before Food	Unhealthy Response	Healthy Response

☞ *Tools for action*

You have come to the end of Step 5 where we have helped you to *become aware of your triggers*. Here is a reminder of what you need to do:

√ When feeling hungry, determine whether you are physically or psychologically hungry and have a healthy response strategy in place.

√ Become aware of the thoughts, emotions and situations which trigger you to overeat.

√ Feelings of fear can dictate how we eat. Become aware of your food fears, e.g., do you avoid eating in the company of others? The best strategy in coping with such fears is not avoidance but gradual exposure – gently place yourself to face up to whatever you are afraid of, e.g., eating in the company of others.

√ Everyday choices determine long-term success at weight loss. Record your eating patterns in your *triggers table* for one week and find out if your responses to food triggers are healthy or unhealthy.

I wanted to keep losing weight my secret, but I soon discovered I needed the support of family and friends – when I felt like giving up, it was their words of encouragement that helped me to go on.

STEP 6

HAVE THE COURAGE TO REACH OUT FOR HELP

10

Sharing Your Dream

I am part of all that I have met.

– Tennyson

The power of people support can never be underestimated. Where would the greatest team in the world be without their supporters rooting for them, cheering them on? People are one of our most important resources when we are taking on a new challenge – we need cheerleaders in our corner, encouraging and supporting us all the way.

Have a think about the most significant people in your life – those you feel closest to. Are you prepared to share your weight loss dreams with them? If not, what is stopping you? Could it be for any of the following reasons?

(a) You have poor self-esteem and prefer not to disclose your deepest desires to others.

People who lack self-esteem find it difficult to accept that other people love them for who they are. Because you do not accept yourself unconditionally, you can't imagine why other people would. Building up relationships with others will help you learn to love yourself as you are and accept that other people love you too – accepting this is a real self-esteem booster.

(b) You don't want to appear vulnerable in front of others.

Do you go around wearing the mask of success – pretending that you are successful at everything all the time and afraid that one day, somebody is going to see through you and catch you out? Such zeal to be perfect is incredibly stressful – which of us is successful at everything we do? Long-lasting relationships are based on honesty, we feel comfortable revealing ourselves to others and, in turn, receive much satisfaction from the knowledge that we are loved and accepted even when we do fail. So, tell your loved ones you need their help and support and they will be happy to give it. Living free from the mask of success will be truly liberating.

(c) Your pride is holding you back from being dependant on others.

Nobody wants to be a relationship leech – someone who is all the time trying to please other people, seek their approval, and does not want to do anything on their own. This type of relationship is completely one-sided and is not good for either party. Even in our closest relationships, we need to maintain our individuality – a separate space where we have the freedom to be who we are, have friends, hobbies, and interests of our own. On the other hand, some are so independent that they don't want other people involved in their lives in any way. When you completely separate yourself from others, you are depriving yourself of a lot of happiness – just think of all those words of encouragement and comforting hugs you are missing.

Gather up your cheerleaders
√ Tell the important people in your life about your weight loss plans. The decisions you make are most likely going to affect them too, and they will be grateful that you have let them know. They may offer support before you even have to ask, and if they do, accept it.
√ Avoid revealing your plans to people you suspect will not be supportive. Their feedback will not be constructive because it could be motivated by negative emotions such as jealousy or anger.
√ Keep your supporters regularly updated of your progress – tell them about the good and bad times. Ask them for feedback

and listen to what they say because they have your best interests at heart.

√ Be open about your feelings at all times. It's wonderful to know that other people accept you for who you are.

√ Acknowledge the help and support you get from others, and be prepared to give your support to them when they need it. Good relationships are never one-sided – there is lots of give and take.

√ And remember when things go wrong, don't blame others. The choice to lose weight is yours and it is, ultimately, your responsibility to reach your goal.

John's story

It just had got to the stage where I needed to lose weight. I weighed over 17 stone and buying clothes was a complete nightmare. I just had to mix and match jackets and trousers because my waist so large. When I went out to restaurants, I used to complain all the time that the chairs were uncomfortable. I couldn't wait to get home to spread out on my own couch. Now, of course, I know it wasn't the chairs in the restaurant, it was me!

My wife, Trish, mentioned to me once that she thought I needed to lose weight, but I was angry with her for saying it. I said if she loved me she would accept me as I am. I knew deep down that she said it to me because she was worried about me – a few years before I lost weight, I had developed back problems, high blood pressure and high cholesterol levels. I ignored my health problems and continued overeating until one day, I went to the doctor and he gave me an ultimatum – lose weight or be at serious risk of major ill health that would shorten my life considerably.

I came home and told Trish that I planned to lose weight. It was very difficult telling her about my plans, especially when I had been angry with her before. She was great about it though and told me she would give me every support, and she did. She started to cook low-fat meals, took care of the kids in the evening when I needed to exercise, and just made so many sacrifices so that I could reach my goal. When I put on a few pounds and felt like giving up, she was there to encourage me and she never criticised me or made me feel bad in any way. I could

> not have lost weight without her, she was fantastic. Today I am four stone lighter and my health has improved enormously, my back problems have eased and both blood pressure and cholesterol levels are down – when I went back to the doctor he didn't recognise me! And most important of all, I feel great about myself. I have more energy, I do more things, I enjoy life a whole lot better.

The power of the group

Earlier, we recommended that you join a reputable weight loss class as a way of educating yourself about healthy eating. Another great advantage of being a member of such a class is the support available from the class mentor and members.

The mentor usually has lost weight himself/herself and their personal insights will be of great benefit. As well as support from the mentor, you also meet many other people who, like yourself, are trying to lose weight. Their example, motivational tips and experiences act as a powerful influence; losing weight together is so much easier than doing it on your own. Do not be afraid to let go and speak your mind, you will feel so much better afterwards. With group support, the group acts as your confessor but remember the ground rule of any successful group is that it is non-judgemental.

The following is a diagrammatic representation of sharing your dream in order to achieve your weight loss goal:

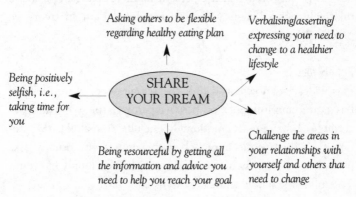

Asking others to be flexible regarding healthy eating plan

Verbalising/asserting/ expressing your need to change to a healthier lifestyle

Being positively selfish, i.e., taking time for you

SHARE YOUR DREAM

Being resourceful by getting all the information and advice you need to help you reach your goal

Challenge the areas in your relationships with yourself and others that need to change

Forgiveness of yourself and others

Life is full of endless opportunities but sometimes we miss out on them because we are still living in the past and worrying about things we did wrong or bad things that happened to us. Take a good look at how you are living and see how we can let go of issues you feel guilty about. Louise L. Hay in her book, *You Too Can Heal Your Life*, talks a lot about forgiveness and letting go of hurts and wrongs done to us.

Make peace with yourself and your past by writing a letter to yourself. Use this letter to talk about the negative emotions you feel and the negative events you have experienced. At first, this may seem strange (writing to yourself), but once you start, you will be surprised at how effective setting your thoughts and feelings down on paper is. Let this letter be your way of forgiving yourself and others for the bad things that have happened, and making peace with yourself.

Resentments may be another reason why you won't achieve your goal or why you won't even ask for help. Before moving towards your final goal, list any resentments you may still have in your life. Do not be afraid to even admit that you resent or perhaps are jealous of somebody else's speed of weight loss.

As a symbol of a final letting go of guilt and resentments, burn the letter and decide that from today, you will enjoy each day to the full, living in the present moment, choosing to eat a relatively normal diet, with the occasional built in treats we previously mentioned.

Family factors

It is widely acknowledged that the happiness of our childhood has a profound influence on how we perceive the world and, accordingly, how we react emotionally as adults. As part of Dr Moore-Groarke's therapeutic approach with families, she usually asks patients to discuss their relationships with their family of origin. The following family traits are discussed:

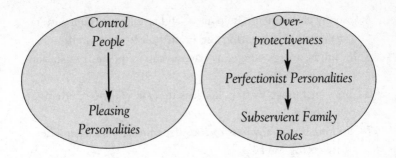

Was your family a controlling one – did you always feel you had to please other people and that your own needs were not taken care of?

Was your family over-protective – were you given the freedom to express yourself as you are, or did you feel you had to live up to people's expectations?

Did you feel an equal member of your family, or were other members considered more important to you?

All of the above family traits are destructive and often lead to negative patterns around food. When looking at your family of origin and how it has moulded you emotionally, it's also a good idea to examine hereditary factors by identifying anybody with a weight or addiction problem. If a member of your family has worked on his/her addictive personality, it might be useful talk with them. Do not be afraid to do this.

Examine your relationships
Take a moment to consider the quality of your relationships with yourself and those around you. Here are some questions to help you focus on your relationships and how you can improve them:

1 What is my relationship like with myself?
2 Who is my significant other, and how do we relate?
3 How can my friends help, for example going walking or exercising with me?

4 Can my children also help me? Can I re-educate them with regard to healthy eating and limit their treats as well?

5 If I am at an age where my parents can help, can I make suggestions to them?

6 Can I encourage work colleagues to walk with me perhaps at lunchtime?

7 Can I encourage my boss to consider canteen menus or a healthy eating week?

Food the pacifier

We have discussed physical versus psychological hunger, pointing out that we often eat when troubled and seeking comfort. Food, on these occasions, acts an emotional crutch or pacifier – it gives us a temporary, short-lived escape from our negative emotions.

In our relationships, food usually acts as a pacifier when it acts as a substitute for the following:

Love	*Touch*	*Sexual Intimacy*	*Comfort*
Support	*Companionship/ friendship*	*Expression of feelings*	

Consider if any of the following apply to you:

Do you overeat because ...

√ You do not love yourself and you do not feel loved.

√ You are not able to cope with stressful conflicts in your relationships.

√ You find it difficult to maintain relationships.

√ You are unable to express your feelings honestly.

√ You are lonely.

√ You miss human contact – getting a big bear hug.

√ You feel isolated because you don't have people around you who support you.

√ You do not enjoy intimate sexual contact.

This is a good time to address the issue of food as a pacifier in our relationships. Significant others will be able to help you see how you use food destructively. If you do not feel comfortable sharing your deepest emotions with someone close to you, seek the help of a professional counsellor. Use the list at the back of this book as a useful guide to some resources. Write and ask for advice and see which one suits you best and, remember, discuss whatever route you decide to take with your doctor first.

You and your significant other
As you embark on your weight loss journey, it is important that your relationship with your significant other is honest and open. It means you can rely on each other for support, but you also have the space to express your individuality. This person's support and positive feedback will be a welcome addition on your journey to weight loss.

The following is a questionnaire Dr Moore-Groarke uses with her clients to assess the quality of relationships with their most significant others. In your notebook, answer the questions as honestly as possible and reflect on what changes you may need to make in your relationships.

1 Do I feel loved/accepted? Do I feel understood/listened to?
2 Am I ever angry with my significant other?
3 Do I have to justify my behaviour?
4 Do I feel inferior?
5 Do I compare myself to this person?
6 Can I rely on this person?
7 Can I speak my mind?
8 Am I assertive with this person?
9 Do I sometimes feel used by this person?

Dos and Don'ts for Relationships Questionnaire

√ If there are areas that need to be addressed, do be prepared to discuss them with your significant other. Have a heart-to-heart, talk about how you feel and share your dreams.

√ Don't blame each other for things that have gone wrong in your relationship, instead use this as an opportunity to build a new, stronger relationship of benefit to both of you.

√ Do listen to what the other person has to say and you will understand them more.

√ Don't lose weight to secure this person's approval, do it for you.

Celebrating your own success with others

If you have achieved some weight loss, treat and reward yourself in the company of other people. Here are some ideas:

- Get a friend to go to the hairdressers with you.
- Join a dancing class.
- Swap a good book.
- Go shopping.
- Go out to the theatre or cinema.
- Plan a holiday.

Homework: Review your contract

Remember the contract you made with yourself at the beginning of Step 2? It's now time to review it and write another contract. This time, get somebody close to you to witness it and date it – their awareness of the promises you make will enable them to support you. Also, the fact that you ask somebody else to witness it indicates that you are ready to make a serious public commitment to lose weight.

When you are writing your contract, include something you have become aware of as you did the exercises in this book. The new contract could go something like this:

I AGREE THAT:

I will lose weight permanently.
I will not let fear stop me from achieving my dream.
I will learn to relax so that I feel less stressed and anxious about dieting.

Signed _____ Dated _____

Witnessed _____ Dated _____

11

Reclaiming Your Rights

We all have rights as individuals but sometimes, due to low self-esteem, we feel that our rights don't really matter, it's more important that other people are pleased. The following is a list of some false assumptions which you may have about how you should act and behave. It's important to confront these assumptions and assert your rights as an individual so that you can choose to lose weight for *you* and nobody else.

1. It is selfish to put your needs before other people's needs versus
You have a right to put yourself first sometimes.

Give yourself the licence to be selfish! And by this, we mean that when it comes to making good choices about how you eat, put your needs first. By taking care of your health, you are reinforcing the belief: I am a worthwhile person. By having the confidence to think of your own needs, you banish memories of unsuccessful attempts at weight loss.

2. It is shameful to make mistakes versus
You have a right to make mistakes.

None of us are perfect – and thank God for that! Nobody has an appropriate response for every occasion. From the beginning of your journey to weight loss, you will need to be prepared for the times you lapse. There will inevitably be times, for one reason or another, when you over indulge. Remember it's not the end of the world. Today is another day, so start over and learn from where you made a mistake. Draw on the ways we are showing you to deal with any negative feelings and thoughts, and pick yourself up. If at first you don't succeed try and try again.

3. If you can't convince others that your feelings are reasonable, then they must be wrong or maybe you are going crazy versus
You have a right to be the final judge of your feelings and accept them as legitimate.

This applies to a large extent to looking for support within the family. Encouragement and support will continue to enhance positive self-belief and keep thoughts and emotions in check. Do not let others patronise you by commenting on the amount you eat as this can cause further conflict and rebellious behaviour.

Anyone who successfully loses weight will tell you that having somebody to talk to when struggling with weight loss has helped them to keep going. We don't have to battle alone. However, if for some reason you cannot reach that supporting person on the particular day you feel bad, go to your diary and write your feelings down. When you meet them again, you can share your struggle with them. In doing this, you can be safe in the knowledge that you are managing your stress/anxiety, as well as your weight loss.

4. You should respect the views of others versus
You have a right to have your own opinions and convictions.

While it is always useful to accept advice, at the end of the day you have to make your own escape from the weight trap. Be selective about what advice you take from other people. Often it is good to listen and learn but remember, what works best for one person may not work best for you. When you are feeling vulnerable you allow others to make choices for you, which is not good for your confidence in the long run.

5. You should always try to be logical and consistent versus
You have a right to change your mind or decide on a different course of action.

To date, you have probably tried several quick-fix approaches to weight loss and, while these may work for someone with a very small amount of weight to shed (less than half a stone), they will not work for somebody who has more to lose. Motivation towards weight loss involves the logic of patience. Impatience at our slow weight loss leads us to change our plan of action and eventually give up. Therefore, before you take an eating and exercise plan on board, do your own research. Look for statistics of successful results, and be prepared that if it is a sensible plan, your weight loss will be gradual but much more successful in the long run.

6. You should be flexible and adjust versus
You have a right to protest.

No matter what the situation, you can assert yourself, for example this might apply to eating out, choosing careful options on a menu and not being afraid to ask for your salad without dressing, and so on.

7. You should not interrupt versus
You have a right to interrupt and ask for clarification.

If there are things about your eating plan that you do not understand or are unsure about, it is your right to ask questions and have information clarified. Assert yourself and you will benefit in the long run.

8. Don't rock the boat versus
You have a right to negotiate change.

Change and adaptation is a common theme throughout this book. Begin by getting rid of words like 'I have to' and 'I should' and replace them with 'I choose to'. Empower yourself to move towards change. Choice leads to positive change as opposed to negative change. When we think about eating healthily in terms of something we want to do rather than something we must do, we are proactive in our own recovery.

For example, when we no longer think or use language such as 'I have to go for a walk' but say 'I choose to go for a walk', we are taking control of the situation and eliminating stress and anxiety. Telling ourselves that we should do this, that or the other creates stress – it's like pushing a boulder up a hill all on our own and it just keeps rolling back down again. Take that weight off your shoulders!

9. *You shouldn't take up people's valuable time with your problems versus* You have a right to ask for help or emotional support.

Reach out to a professional if there are issues or life events that need to be addressed. All too often, those who need to talk the most act as a sponge for other people's problems, thus putting their own needs on hold almost indefinitely.

10. *Be modest when complimented versus* You have a right to receive formal recognition for your hard work and achievements.

Compliments are a great way of helping us continue on our journey. Accept them graciously, but beware of becoming too relaxed and returning to old behaviour patterns.

☞ *Tools for action*

In Step 4 we have asked you to *have the courage to reach out for help*. Here is a reminder of what you need to do:

√ If you find it difficult to share your weight loss dreams with others, identify why and decide today to seek other people's support on your journey.

√ Join a reputable weight loss class, learn from the experience of the mentor and draw on the power of group support.

√ Examine your relationships and reflect on how they can be strengthened.

√ Let go of guilt and resentments and make peace with yourself and others.

√ In your relationships, does food act as an emotional crutch? Do you use it to as a substitute for feeling loved?

√ Understand how your family of origin has influenced you emotionally. Also, examine any hereditary influences regarding health.

√ Don't forget to celebrate your success with others!

√ Every human being has rights, and so do you. Don't let other people's mistaken assumptions and the language of 'should' and 'must' rule your life. Instead, opt for the language of 'choice' and assert your rights.

Since I lost weight, I feel so much better about myself. I am doing more things I enjoy. I have much more confidence. I just feel like a different person inside and out.

STEP 7

DISCOVER WHO YOU REALLY ARE

12

Creating a new life

I was so much older then, I'm younger than that now.
BOB DYLAN

In Step 1, we introduced the Body Mass Index chart to give you an indication of what is a healthy weight for you. We also recommended that you sought medical advice before setting your target weight. Achieving this target will bring immense change to your life, not just to the physical shape of your body, but to your health and general well-being, and this, in turn, will enhance the overall quality of your life.

In recognising this ripple effect, we take a multi-disciplinary approach and consider the many aspects of your life that is influenced by your weight loss. In this chapter, for example, we explore issues such as sleep patterns, stress, exercise, and so on, to help you understand that changing your diet is just one aspect of losing weight successfully. This way, you are much more than an individual with a weight problem and a set of walking symptoms, your life – the person you are, what you do, how you live – are essential elements of your weight loss programme.

The following is a diagrammatic representation of how weight loss and well-being affects many areas of our lives.

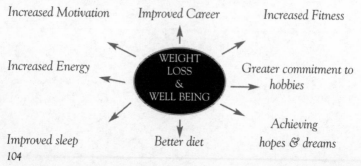

This diagram shows what life is like without weight loss and well being.

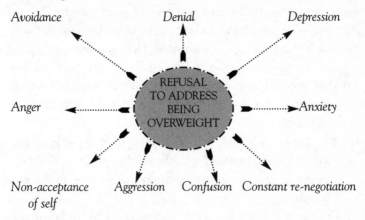

Avoidance   *Denial*   *Depression*

Anger   REFUSAL TO ADDRESS BEING OVERWEIGHT   *Anxiety*

Non-acceptance of self   *Aggression*   *Confusion*   *Constant re-negotiation*

Holistic programme of wellness

As well as starting to eat healthily, begin to take care of other areas of your life so that your weight loss programme is a Holistic Programme of Wellness. Here are some examples of lifestyle changes you can make:

1. Strike a balance between work and play

The old saying that too much work makes Jack a dull boy is very true, however these days many of us find our lives consumed by work, with the result that stress is too common.

Stress can be caused by:

(a) unrealistic expectations of ourselves – trying to do everything and be everything to everybody ...

(b) fear of change and fear of failure – will I be able to cope?...

(c) poor time management – too much to do and not enough time to do it ...

(d) looking on the bleak side of things – what if something goes wrong? ...

Learn to deal with stress by identifying what causes it, then tackling it gradually and realistically. Don't be tempted to try to change everything instantly because this type of gung-ho attitude can turn out to be stressful in its own right! Little by little you will become better with coping with stress. Here are some tips:

(a) Pace yourself at work by making a list of your daily tasks. Prioritise what you need to do today and what can wait until tomorrow.

(b) You simply can't be everything to everybody. If you have too many demands made of you, the result is pressure. Build up your self-esteem by learning to say 'no' to some of the demands.

(c) Do your best but if you don't succeed, don't be hard on yourself. Your life is not intended to be a pressure cooker!

(d) Stop rushing! You might say, but I need to rush because I have so much to do! There are 24 hours in every day, consider if you use them well. If you start your day in a hurry, chances are you will feel stressed before you even get to work. Why not get up thirty minutes earlier and give yourself time to sit down over breakfast? It's a small change but you will be amazed at the difference it makes to your day.

(e) If your desk is untidy or your house is upside down, you will feel less in control. A little bit of time invested in tidying or cleaning every day will keep things running smoothly. This way you won't feel overwhelmed when you can't find a document that's buried under a pile of paperwork or you have visitors coming in an hour and you need to clean your house now!

(f) Avoid making rules for yourself. Instead of telling yourself you 'should' go on a diet, tell yourself that it would be worthwhile to go on a diet. This way you are choosing to go on a diet, not doing so because you feel you have to. If we feel we have to do something, we are already putting ourselves under too much pressure. As we said before, when we do something out of choice, we are making an informed decision and we are in control.

(g) Exercise regularly and find ways to relax and switch off. Have lots of time for yourself every week and you will discover that you have, in turn, lots more to give other people.

(h) Combine healthy eating with some form of relaxation therapy such as visualisation, yoga or meditation. If you feel you need medication, find out about homeopathic alternatives to traditional anxiolytic (anxiety reducing) medication for reducing stress and anxiety. *Again, always consult your doctor for advice.*

2. Take gentle exercise

Regular, gentle exercise is good for both our physical and mental health.

√ It both protects against stress and alleviates it.

√ It is good for our hearts and our circulation in general.

√ It makes dieting easier and when we reach our goal will help us to stay there for life, if we continue to combine gentle exercise with our healthy eating pattern.

√ It strengthens our breathing.

√ It tones our figures and gives our skin a healthy glow.

√ It can improve our social lives if we exercise in a group.

√ It gives us the opportunity to take time out.

√ It helps us feel better generally and improves our energy levels.

If you haven't exercised in a long time, you may not know where to start. Walking is a popular first choice. All you need to do is invest in a good pair walking shoes or runners and wear some loose fitting clothing. Then just walk out the door! You can walk alone or with a friend and one great bonus is that you will be spending time in the outdoors.

If you like to exercise in a group, there are whole lot of other exercises you can try. If you prefer to have a tailor-made exercise programme devised for you, the local gym will be able to help you out. You may try a few different forms of exercise before you find the one you really enjoy.

Note: always consult your doctor for advice before you embark on an exercise programme.

3. Get a good night's sleep

We all need rest and sleep that is not fitful or disturbed. We don't need to sleep perfectly every night but frequent sleepless or restless nights can take their toll. When aiming for a good night's sleep, remember that it is quality of sleep not quantity that's important. While 7–8 hours sleep is regarded as ideal, if we sleep well for less, we will still feel refreshed in the morning.

If you have difficulty sleeping, here are some tips:

√ Only go to bed when you feel tired.
√ Try to get up at the same time every day, this way your sleep routine will be better.
√ Avoid caffeine or alcohol before bedtime. Opt for a calming cup of camomile tea.
√ If you feel peckish before bedtime, have a light snack. Never have a heavy meal.
√ After a hard day, wind down before going to bed by having a lukewarm lavender bath.
√ Never work in your bedroom. Your mind needs to associate your bedroom with rest and relaxation.

4. Cut out cigarettes and have alcohol in moderation

The effects that smoking and passive smoking have on our health are well documented. In spite of this, many are afraid to give up cigarettes in case they put on weight. The good news is that it is possible to give up cigarettes and lose weight, particularly if you have the support of a good weight loss programme. Giving up cigarettes is difficult but it will be worth the effort for your health.

Likewise, a heavy consumption of alcohol is detrimental to health. It also is the cause of many social problems such as violence on the streets and in the home. A glass of wine in moderation is enjoyable but it's a good idea to bear in mind the negative effects of drinking too much, including the fact that alcohol leads to weight gain.

5. Nourish your spirit

Think of something you really enjoy doing. When you're doing it, you are unaware of time and you have a special feeling inside. By this special feeling, we mean that you get a sense of peace and tranquillity, the type of emotion that many experience when they look at a sunset or see something beautiful in nature.

If you know something that makes you feel this way, take time out at least once a week to do it. If you can't think of anything, try to find something you think you would enjoy. You may not find it on your first attempt but by searching you will get there. For some people, it is reading a book or painting a picture or having a massage. Whatever works for you do it and you will be nourishing a place deep inside of you that helps you feel relaxed and at peace with yourself and the world.

6. Look your best

When the cost of living is high, going to the hairdressers or buying clothes is regarded as a luxury. However, try to budget a little money every month for taking care of your appearance. It might be an idea to put aside the money you save from not buying biscuits and cakes or by not smoking and use this for a visit to the hairdressers or beauticians. When we take care of our appearance, we are giving ourselves the thumbs-up. We are saying to ourselves, 'I like you. You are worthwhile.'

7. Break out of your comfort zone

In Chapter 5, we spoke about how uncomfortable our comfort zone can be! Make a point of regularly challenging your fears. If your fear is of flying, then go on a foreign holiday. If your fear is of heights, then take that lift to the top floor and enjoy the view. The bottom line is that a life lived in fear is a life half-lived. Face your fears and you will get the rewards.

8. Give a helping hand.

Those who bring sunshine to the lives of others cannot keep it from themselves – JAMES M. BARRIE

It's very easy to get wrapped up in our own concerns. One way of counter-acting a tendency to self-obsess is to give a little time each week to doing something useful for another person.

Some of the advantages of sharing our skills free of charge are:

√ You improve your social contact and possibly make new friends.
√ You feel good about yourself because you are doing something worthwhile.
√ You feel satisfied when you see the results of your work.
√ You become aware that life does not just revolve around you and your worries.

We recommend one hour voluntary work a week. Is there an elderly neighbour who needs their shopping done? Maybe you could help out at the local charity shop? Is the local youth club looking for voluntary help? Here are some tips for helping other people:

√ Only offer help to people who seek it. Never impose yourself on people who do not want your help, no matter how good your intentions are.

√ Offer practical help in a non-judgemental manner. Nobody wants others to feel sorry for them, so don't let the person feel you are helping them out of pity.

√ Make it clear that you enjoy helping the other person. It is a two-way transaction, both people benefit. Therefore, they are not indebted to you.

√ Don't try to take the other person's problems on board. You are there just to help them a little. Be clear that you can't help them with everything and never let them manipulate you into feeling guilty if you are unable to meet all their demands.

√ Always keep in mind the reason why you are offering help. It is not an ego trip but an attempt to share your skills to benefit other people.

9. *Live for the moment*

If you spend a lot of time worrying about will happen and feeling bad about what did happen, then you are wasting a lot of energy and causing yourself unnecessary heartache. Put things in perspective by living for the moment because that's all any of us have anyway. None of us know what is going to happen in the future or, indeed, how long our future will be. If we could really appreciate the now, we would be living full and happy lives. Again, human nature being what it is, we won't remember to do this all of the time, but it's certainly worth striving for some of the time.

PROMISE YOURSELF

The key to permanent weight loss is permanent lifestyle changes. It's tempting to go on a 'miracle' diet and lose weight instantly but the truth is, you will put it back on just as quickly. This is due to two reasons: you did not embark on a sensible healthy eating programme, and you have not put the necessary lifestyle changes in place to maintain your weight loss in the long term.

So promise yourself now to make some lifestyle changes. Here are some examples:

√ *I will take a break from the office at lunchtime and go for a walk.*
√ *I will walk up the stairs instead of taking the lift.*
√ *I will go to a weight loss class and educate myself about low-fat food alternatives.*
√ *I will ask my friend to go for a gentle walk with me in the evenings.*
√ *I will get ideas for cooking from a healthy cookbook.*
√ *I will take time to enjoy my meals every day.*
√ *I will take time for myself, if only a few minutes, every day.*
√ *I will make a weekly date in my diary with myself to do something I really enjoy.*

Homework: Lifestyle quiz

Take a few minutes to do this quiz and see if it helps pinpoint the aspects of your lifestyle that need to be changed. Please note: the conclusions are not definitive but act only as a guide.

1. I drive to the corner shop.
     (a) Always   ☐
     (b) Sometimes   ☐
     (c) Never   ☐

2. When my children don't eat their dinner, I eat their leftovers even if I've had my own dinner.
- (a) Always ☐
- (b) Sometimes ☐
- (c) Never ☐

3. I exercise three times a week.
- (a) Always ☐
- (b) Sometimes ☐
- (c) Never ☐

4. I am so tired in the evenings that I eat convenience foods.
- (a) Always ☐
- (b) Sometimes ☐
- (c) Never ☐

5. I put lots of effort into finding out about cooking low fat food.
- (a) Always ☐
- (b) Sometimes ☐
- (c) Never ☐

6. I really enjoy my meals and take time savouring my food.
- (a) Always ☐
- (b) Sometimes ☐
- (c) Never ☐

7. I am constantly juggling work, family and other chores.
- (a) Always ☐
- (b) Sometimes ☐
- (c) Never ☐

Scores per questions:

Question 1:
(a) 15
(b) 10
(c) 5
Question 2:
(a) 15
(b) 10
(c) 5
Question 3:
(a) 5
(b) 10
(c) 15
Question 4:
(a) 15

(b) 10
(c) 5
Question 5:
(a) 5
(b) 10
(c) 15
Question 6:
(a) 5
(b) 10
(c) 15
Question 7:
(a) 15
(b) 10
(c) 5

Your results
Scored 81 – 105
Your lifestyle is most likely holding you back from being a healthy weight. Start by making some small changes and you will see the benefits of healthy eating, being more active and less stressed.

Scored 61 – 80
You are probably leading a reasonably healthy life with room for improvement. Look at the areas where you can improve your eating and exercise habits and take better care of yourself.

Scored 35 – 60
Well done! It looks like you are conscious of what you eat and how much you exercise, and you are taking care of your needs. The result is your body and mind are reaping the rewards.

13

Staying Slim for Life

Successful weight loss is about learning from the past, freeing ourselves from the chains of the past, and creating a better future for ourselves where we have the freedom to be the person we really are. Losing weight is not about battling with our bodies, it's about making friends with ourselves, taking care of ourselves, loving ourselves, understanding ourselves and, ultimately, being ourselves. Achieving weight loss can be a wonderful time of awakening, it's why so many people who achieve their goals say that so much more than their weight has changed – they feel like a different person inside.

So in trying to lose weight, you need to consider:

(a) your relationship with yourself and others, and
(b) your relationship with your body.

Many people mistakenly only focus on how they treat their body in terms of diet and exercise and do not consider how they think, feel and react to situations, and how they relate to the world around them. You cannot achieve successful weight loss unless you are prepared to slim both on the inside and outside, unless you are mentally and emotionally ready and have all the support, resources and skills you need to get to your goal.

As stated earlier, miracle diets sound wonderful and can have amazing short-term results, but what use are they if they do not help you stay slim for the rest of your life? They only serve to prolong your battle with your weight problem because they do not educate you about healthy eating and do not give you the support you need. On the other hand, people who successfully lose weight often say that they finally did it because they were 'ready'. They may have been eternal Monday morning dieters in the past, tried all sorts of dieting gimmicks, and even embarked on reputable healthy eating programmes, but nothing worked until deep inside, they knew they had the resources to cope with the challenge of weight loss and the hurdles they would inevitably have to climb.

So, there are a number of ground rules when trying to achieve a healthy eating lifestyle.

1 You need to be mentally and emotionally ready before you start. In other words, you need to believe that you can do it, that you are worthwhile.
2 You need to be able to stick to your healthy eating plan. This means that when you lapse along the way, you will be able to pick yourself up and get going again.
3 You need to have a time frame that is realistic. As we pointed out previously, a healthy weight loss plan aims to help you lose one to two pounds per week.
4 You need to make informed choices. Find out what you need to do to succeed by exploring the options available to you and then deciding which one suits you best.
5 You need to want success. If you are not motivated, you will find it a struggle to keep going.

How have you been doing?
Now is a good time to assess how much you have achieved since starting to read this book. Maybe you have decided to go along to your local weight loss class, maybe you have already started to lose weight, or maybe you haven't made any progress yet. If you haven't started to change yet, then the time may not have yet been right for you.

√ Do out a new goal plan. Write down your short-term and long-term goals. New goals must be realistic, positive, achievable, and can be maintained.

√ Redo your contract with yourself and be clear about what you hope to achieve.

√ Accept yourself as you are and decide to lose weight out of love for yourself.

√ Let go of past failures.

√ Make a positive choice for you by starting your weight loss journey today, not tomorrow, not next Monday morning.

√ Live in the here and now.

√ Embrace your life and enjoy it – there's no point in living complaining.

Ask yourself:

1　What do I hope to achieve?
2　What steps am I going to take?
3　How will I assess my programme?
4　How could I choose to sabotage my weight loss plan?
5　How will I avoid possible sabotage?
6　How will I reward myself for achieving short-term goals?
7　When will I celebrate achieving my final long-term goal?

When you set out to achieve a personal goal, it's easy to feel excited and enthusiastic in the beginning, however many lose such heady feelings on encountering the first obstacle that comes their way.

In order to overcome obstacles and recover quickly from relapses, you need to:

• Be flexible. Accept that neither you nor the world around is perfect. Therefore, it's okay not to get everything right all the time.

- Don't blame yourself. Understand that your relapse is not due to a character flaw but is due to something such as the fact you are under a lot of stress of late. Learning why you re-lapse will enable you to put a mechanism in place to avoid the same pitfall again.
- Give yourself lots of time to get to a goal. Establishing a goal hierarchy will help you take smaller, achievable steps along the way.
- Acknowledge successes. It's easy to discount achievements if you have not reached your goal yet, but remember that every step you take is closer to your goal. So give yourself a regular clap on the back and tell yourself how great you are.
- Educate yourself about stress and identify ways you can reduce it in your life.
- Get all the information, resources and skills you need. This may mean going to a weight loss class, seeking the advice of a nutritionist, or attending a counsellor. Whatever you need to do, do it because it will be worth it in the end.
- Continue to hope. No matter how many times you lapse along the way, you can achieve your goal if you stay focused and believe you can do it.
- Dream about being slim. Visualise how you would look and what you would do differently if you were slim. Let this mental image keep you going when you are feeling low.

Step by step out of the weight trap
You may be reading this and still feeling stuck in the weight trap. If so, there are a number of steps you can take to help you con-front this destructive pattern of living.

1 Understand that you need to lose weight for your health's sake. See your doctor on a regular basis for a medical check-up.
2 Keep a diary of your thoughts and feelings. Mood swings lead to overeating. If your experience frequent mood swings, it

is advisable to talk to your GP for advice because you may
be depressed.

3 Do not be afraid to get a second opinion regarding your weight
management. Often it is necessary to seek help and support
from a number of different professionals, such as a nutritionist, GP, psychologist, and so on.

4 Having a mentor is a good strategy. Remember you do not need
to have a psychological problem to go for counselling.

5 Set specific changes as your goals but be realistic regarding such
changes. Don't expect too much too soon.

6 Explore all possible pitfalls which cause you stress and anxiety.
Identify these difficulties in your work, home, family, and
social life and develop a strategy for reducing stress.

7 Ask your spouse, partner, children or friends to help you with
your fight-back plan.

8 Have a realistic time scale in place to achieve your goals.

9 Contract to follow your life changes plan for a set period, for
example three months, and then review.

10 With regard to lifestyle changes, keep adapting your approach
until you get what you want.

When you reach your goal weight, the next step is learning to
maintain your new weight. Being slim is a choice you will need
to make every day for the rest of your life. You can do this by com-
bining a healthy balanced diet with regular gentle exercise. Keep
up your motivation by having a cut-off point beyond which you
will not put on any more weight – many weight loss organisations
use this method to ensure that their members do not pile on the
pounds all over again. Say your target weight is $9^1/_2$ stone, then
make a decision that if you reach 10 stone, you will begin your
weight loss plan again.

Ultimately, by accepting that you are worthwhile as a person, that you deserve to enjoy good health and happiness as much
as anybody else, you will be able to achieve weight loss and keep

it off for the rest of your life. We are inviting you to a better quality of life, better mental, emotional and physical health.

The choice is yours. Which is easier to choose?:

The pleasure of being free to express yourself, to be the person you really are

or

The pain of being stuck in the weight trap, trapped by negative thoughts, emotions and behaviour?

If you choose freedom and change, we wish you every success. Let your weight loss journey be your opportunity to discover the real you and to embrace every opportunity for happiness and peace.

☞ *Tools for action*

Congratulations, you have completed the final step of your weight loss plan. Here is a reminder of Step 7, where we helped you to *discover who you really are*, together with a final check before you proceed with the rest of your weight loss journey:

√ As part of your Holistic Programme of Wellness, become aware of the lifestyle changes you need to make to get to your goal and stay there.

√ Understand that refusal to address your weight problem is not an option if you want to lead a healthy, fulfilled life.

√ Calculate your total weight loss so far. Give yourself credit for everything you have achieved.

√ How far are you from your desired weight? As before, break down the next part of your journey into achievable goals.

√ Examine your food diaries and re-read your written exercises. Sometimes we need to hear and read things many times before we are finally able to take them on board.

√ Have you discovered an exercise you enjoy?

√ Use your weight loss journey as a time to discover inner peace.

√ Do you need support? If you haven't got the support of friend or family or a weight loss organisation yet, now is a good time to get it.

√ You are embarking on a process of personal change which will create new opportunities for you in the future. Have a long-term plan. Keep in mind that your plan to lose weight is for life, therefore the lifestyle changes you put in place now need to be long-lasting.

√ Always remember you are worthwhile as a person and you deserve to enjoy good health and happiness.

Appendix

Useful Names and Addresses

The following is a list of names and addresses you may find useful, together with a brief outline of the function of each one. It is advisable to contact your general practitioner first, and s/he may be able to provide you with information on medical professionals or sources of help in your local area.

Dr G. Moore-Groarke, Suite 21, Cork Clinic, Western Road, Cork. Registered Consultant Psychologist with special interest in the area of eating disorders, health psychology, child and adolescent problems pain and stress management. Also health advisor to Weight Watchers Ireland. Telephone/ fax: 021–4343073 or log on to: www.corkclinic.com

Weight Watchers Ireland, 1 Phibsboro Road, Dublin 7. Leading weight loss organisation with over 900 classes held weekly nationwide. Low call: 1850 234 123 or log on to: www.weightwatchers.com. For information on classes in Northern Ireland, telephone 028 90426812/ 028 86766330

Eating Disorder Unit, St Patrick's hospital, James Street, Dublin 8. Largest inpatient unit in Ireland for the treatment of the eating disorders anorexia nervosa and bulimia. Telephone: 01–2493200 or log onto: www.stpatrickshosp.com

Overeaters Anonymous, PO Box 2529, Dublin 5. Offers a programme of recovery from compulsive overeating using the Twelve Steps and Twelve Traditions of Overeaters Anonymous. Telephone: 01–2788106

BodyWhys, Central Office, PO Box 105, Blackrock, Co. Dublin. Irish national charity which offers help, support and understanding for people with eating disorders, their families and friends. Telephone/ fax: 01-2834963 or call confidential helpline: 01–2835126 or log on to: www.bodywhys.ie

Irish Medical Directory, PO Box 5049, Dublin 6. Comprehensive and widely used guide to health care and the medical profession in Ireland. Telephone: 01–4926040 or log on to: www.imd.ie

Irish Society of Homeopaths, 35-37 Dominick St, Galway. Representative body of professional homeopaths in Ireland. Telephone/fax:

091– 565040 or log on to: www.irishsocietyofhomeopaths.com

Irish Association for Counselling & Therapy, 8 Cumberland Street, Dun Laoghaire, Co. Dublin. Establishes, maintains and regulates standards for the profession of counselling and therapy in Ireland. Telephone: 01–2300061 or log on to: www.irish-counselling.ie

Psychological Society of Ireland, CX House, 2A Corn Exchange Place, Dublin 2. Professional body for psychologists in Ireland which aims to advance psychology as a pure and applied science in Ireland and elsewhere. Telephone/fax: 01–6717122

The British Psychological Society, St Andrews House, 48 Princess Road East, Leicester LE1 7DR. Representative body for psychologists and psychology in the UK. Telephone: 0044 116 254 9568/ fax 0044 116 247 0787/ or log on to: www.bps.org.uk

Irish Patients Association Ltd., Unit 1, First Floor, 24 Church Road, Ballybrack, Co. Dublin. Aims to place the patient at the centre of health care, improve the quality and service they receive, improve the cost effectiveness, improve the availability of service and protect present and future patients' rights. Telephone: 01–2722555 or log on to: www.irishpatients.ie

The above list is published for information purposes only. As not all forms of treatment are suitable for everyone, it would be prudent and advisable to consult with a general practitioner before embarking on any course of treatment. *Please note:* Dr G. Moore-Groarke does not accept patients without a referral letter from a general practitioner or medical consultant.

Progress Chart

We have given you an example of a completed Progress Chart. In the bottom left-hand corner of the chart, the starting weight is recorded. In Week 1, the person lost 2 pounds, while in Week 3, the person gained 2 pounds. By the end of week 7, the person had lost 8 pounds.

Points to note:
- Only record your weight once a week. Ignore daily weight fluctuations – it's your weight loss over the week that counts. For long-term success, we recommend a gradual loss of 1 – 2 pounds per week.
- Be realistic – you will not lose weight every week. You, more than likely, will put a few pounds on some weeks due to special celebrations such as birthdays, physical set-backs such as colds and flu, stresses such as work commitments, and so on. Life doesn't always go smoothly – don't expect your weight loss to go smoothly either! The important thing is not to give up but always pick yourself up and start again.
- When assessing your progress, concentrate on the big picture. Don't worry about the weeks you didn't lose weight. Focus instead on the overall result over, for example, four weeks and then you will see how much you've really achieved.
- I f you have had a successful week, try to identify what helped with the weight loss; equally, identify on a bad week what held back your weight loss.

EXAMPLE OF PROGRESS CHART

	Week 1	Week 2	Week 3	Week 4	Week 5	Week 6	Week 7
9 st 2lb							
12 lb							
10 lb							
8 lb							
6 lb							
4lb							
2lb							
10 st 2lb							
12 lb							
10 lb							
8 lb							
6lb							
4 lb							
2 lb							
11 st 2 lb							
12lb							
10 lb							
8 lb						●	●
6 lb					●		
4 lb		●		●			
2 lb	●		●				
12 st 2 lb							

Week	1	2	3	4	5	6	7

My Progress Chart

St lb							
12 lb							
10 lb							
8 lb							
6 lb							
4lb							
2lb							
St lb							
12 lb							
10 lb							
8 lb							
6lb							
4 lb							
2 lb							
st lb							
12 lb							
10 lb							
8 lb							
6 lb							
4 lb							
2 lb							
St lb							

Put your starting weight here

| Week | 1 | 2 | 3 | 4 | 5 | 6 | 7 |

Recommended Reading

If you are looking for further reading on your weight loss journey, you may find the following books helpful. We list them here under relevant subjects.

Negative Thinking

Burns, David D. MD, *The Feeling Good Handbook*, Plume/Penguin, 1989
Greenberger, Dennis, Ph.D & Padesky, Christine A. PhD, *Mind Over Mood – Change How You Feel by Changing the Way You Think*, The Guilford Press, 1995

Fear

Jeffers, Susan, *Feel the Fear and Do It Anyway, How to Turn Your Fear and Indecision into Confidence and Action*, Arrow Books, 1991
Peiffer, Vera, *Positively Fearless*, Element, 1993
Spindler, Stéphanie, *Learn to Live – The Key to Unlocking Your True Potential*, Element, 1991

Stress

Claus, Karen E. & Bailey, June T., *Living with Stress and Promoting Well-Being*, The C.V. Mosby Company, 1980
Keane, Colm, *The Stress File*, RTE Blackwater Press, 1997
Madders, Jane, *The Stress and Relaxation Handbook – A Practical Guide to Self Help Techniques*, Vermillion, 1979
Markham, Ursula, *Managing Stress – The Practical Guide to Using Stress Positively*, Element, 1989

Spirit

Albom, Mitch, *Tuesdays with Morrie*, Little, Brown and Company, 1997
De Mello, Anthony, *Walking on Water – Reaching God in Our Time*, The Columba Press, 1998
Hay, Louise, *You Too Can Heal Your Life*, Hay House, 1989

More Interesting Books

WHEN FOOD BECOMES YOUR ENEMY
Gillian Moore-Groarke and Sylvia Thompson

Anorexia, bulimia and comfort eating have become serious problems, with many families having to cope with the trauma of a son
or daughter suffering from an eating disorder.

When Food Becomes Your Enemy explains simply how anorexia,
bulimia or comfort eating can take over your life and why any eating
problem is really only a symptom of deeper unease within the person

Case histories illustrate the painful process from the initial stages
to recovery, with sufferers illuminating in an honest way what is really
going on when food becomes your enemy.

DREAMING WITH TONY DE MELLO
A Handbook of Meditation Exercises

John Callanan, SJ

This book illustrates some of the central themes of De Mello's life
and vision and explains how De Mello ran his prayer workshops and
fantasy exercises. It also contains prayer exercises, gospel meditations
and fantasy style prayer, created by John Callanan, based on the style
made popular by De Mello.

BEYOND PROZAC
Healing Mental Suffering without Drugs

Dr Terry Lynch

In this controversial, deeply felt and hard-hitting book, Terry Lynch
takes issue with conventional medical treatment of psychiatric or
emotional illness. He questions how doctors diagnose different levels
of emotional disturbance and the efficacy – and inherent dangers –
of the drug therapies that are offered to many people as a matter of
course.